Nutritional Counseling *for* Lifestyle Change

Nutritional Counseling *for* Lifestyle Change

Linda Snetselaar

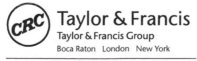

Taylor & Francis
Taylor & Francis Group
Boca Raton   London   New York

CRC is an imprint of the Taylor & Francis Group,
an informa business

Press
r & Francis Group
Broken Sound Parkway NW, Suite 300
Raton, FL 33487-2742

7 by Taylor and Francis Group, LLC
Press is an imprint of Taylor & Francis Group, an Informa business

aim to original U.S. Government works
ed in the United States of America on acid-free paper
765432

national Standard Book Number-10: 0-8493-1604-9 (Hardcover)
national Standard Book Number-13: 978-0-8493-1604-3 (Hardcover)
ry of Congress Card Number 2006044026

Library of Congress Cataloging-in-Publication Data

Snetselaar, Linda G.
   Nutrition counseling for lifestyle change / Linda Snetselaar.
      p. cm.
   Includes bibliographical references and index.
   ISBN 0-8493-1604-9 (alk. paper)
    1. Nutrition counseling. 2. Health counseling. 3. Obesity--Psychological
aspects. I. Title.

RC628S642 2006
616.3'9806--dc22   2006044026

the Taylor & Francis Web site at
//www.taylorandfrancis.com

he CRC Press Web site at
//www.crcpress.com

PREFACE

This book is a combination of experiences in which I have been involved over my professional career. It brings a combination of ideas together that include methods of communicating, strategies for behavior change, ways to assess problems, and methods to facilitate self-management. The concepts presented in this book have been tested in a variety of clinical trials where lifestyle change was needed to determine if dietary change affected disease.

The goal of lifestyle change as presented here is to maximize the patients' abilities to tailor a strategy to their current situation and make a major and lasting change that improves health over time. Sections in this book present ways to facilitate change in different age groups based on clinical trial work.

Examples of dialogues that occur with specific age groups of patients illustrate what might actually happen as counseling for change occurs. Innovative ways of communicating are presented with new strategies for facilitating the patients' ways of dealing with stress as eating habits change.

In general, this is a text for the practitioner and student who strive to help the patient change in a tailored fashion that potentially assures success relative to maintenance.

THE AUTHOR

Linda G. Snetselaar is currently a professor in the Department of Epidemiology, College of Public Health at the University of Iowa. She is an endowed Chair of Preventive Nutrition Education. Her work has been in the area of multi-center randomized clinical trials mostly funded by the National Institutes of Health and emphasizing dietary change over long periods of time. She has focused on how to change and maintain eating behaviors with a focus on affecting dietary habits in individuals throughout the United States.

Dr. Snetselaar has been a director of many workshops on the topic of dietary change using an eclectic behaviorally based approach. She has worked to change eating behaviors in a variety of research projects: The Lipid Research Clinics Study, The Diabetes Control and Complications Trial, The Modification of Diet in Renal Disease Study, The Diet Intervention Study in Children, The Diet Intervention Study in Children 2006, The Women's Intervention Nutrition Study, and the Women's Health Initiative. She has also provided expertise to wellness programs for large industries. She is currently focused on translating much of what was learned in these long-term trials to routine care in clinics in the United States.

Dr. Snetselaar teaches master's, doctoral, and medical students in the Colleges of Public Health and Medicine at the University of Iowa. She enjoys facilitating the learning process and being a mentor to students. Dr. Snetselaar is chair of her college's Faculty Council and serves on the University Faculty Senate and Council.

CONTENTS

1

INTRODUCTION

The concept of nutrition lifestyle change as it is described in this text includes not only eating habits but the environmental factors that surround them. Lifestyle change for improved eating patterns is complex. Changes in eating habits require a knowledge of eating patterns and discovery of the role past history played in shaping the way we eat. Additionally, lifestyle change must be based upon behavioral theories as they relate to dietary habit modification. An in-depth awareness of the importance of foods, their nutrient composition, and methods of food preparation should be a focus. Along with emphasis on diet is the immense importance of daily activity and planned exercise. It is beyond the focus of this text to describe specifics related to activity and exercise, but that does not diminish their immense importance in the process of lifestyle change. Equally important is our desire to minimize stress in our lives as lifestyle change occurs. This important concept will be dealt with in discussions related to eating and food preparation.

1.1 THE MEDITERRANEAN DIET AND ITS PAST INFLUENCES

In our American culture we have adopted a love for many ethnic dishes. One of those is the food and beverage characteristics of the Mediterranean diet. This eating pattern is of importance in this book because it includes many topics related to those discussed in the paragraph above. Nestle indicates that the Mediterranean diet is of value as a model of a dietary pattern that results in one of the lowest incidence rates of chronic diseases and highest life expectancies compared to other regions in the world [1–5]. Table 1.1 and Table 1.2 show comparisons of Italian and U.S. life expectancy data.

Table 1.1 Life Expectancy Early 1990s — Italy and the U.S.[a]

	Italy	U.S.
Women	80.5	79.2
Men	73.7	72.2

[a] Australian Institute of Health and Welfare Australia's Health 1996. Canberra. Australian Government Printing Service; 1996.

Table 1.2 Life Expectancy Today — Italy and the U.S.

	Italy	U.S.
Women	82.0	79.4
Men	75.8	73.9

Note: Annuario statisticl italiano–2000. Rome, ISTAT, 2001. OECD health data 2000: a comparative analysis of 29 countries. Paris: Organization for Economic Co-operation and Development, 2000. http://www.cdc.gov/nchs/data/hus/tables/2003/03hus027.pdf.

We learn from a study of the Mediterranean diet that not only are specific foods and beverages important, but a lifestyle of physical activity and attention to reduced stress is also paramount. Love of food in the Mediterranean culture means preparing and eating food in a slow and relaxed fashion. The focus is on enjoying the process of food preparation and then eating slowly to experience flavors, textures, aromas, and colors in each dish.

The Mediterranean diet has an ancient history that provides reasons for the specific foods enjoyed in this eating pattern. To understand why this population living in certain regions bordering the Mediterranean Sea eat in a specific way, we must look back to past centuries and their influence on eating habits.

Evidence of ancient diets in the regions bordering the Mediterranean Sea are in abundance [6]. Nestle indicates the problems in evaluating evidence from a variety of sources. The problems include translating, classifying, dating, and interpreting information. In spite of these difficulties, researchers have documented plant and animal, bread, spices, sweets, beer, and wine from ancient cultures [6–9]. It should be noted that the presence of foods in a region is an association and not firm proof of its usual consumption. Writers of the classics speak of the foods eaten by warriors and noblemen.

Researchers who have carefully analyzed Homer's writings note that the food of this elite group of people included mostly meat, bread, and wine [9]. The common people consumed a diet based on plant foods and bread, with seafood eaten only occasionally. Olive oil was also abundant [9].

From the second to third century, in classical texts, poets describe foods in terms of their flavors, aromas, preparation methods, and their role in everyday meals and elaborate banquets. This might indicate that the Mediterranean diet of the time was consumed by all classes of the Mediterranean populace [10].

Montanari describes two opposing cultures: one based on bread, wine, and oil and the other on meat, milk, and butter [11]. Archaeological studies of human remains found in medieval sites indicate a very balanced diet. The reality in medieval times was that when famine occurred because of drought, other sources of food — lamb, fish, beef, and sheep's milk helped assure adequate nutritional intakes [12]. Montanari presents the differences between peasants and noblemen [13]. Peasants almost always boiled meat dishes. Noblemen roasted meat on long skewers on wide grills. For the warring nobles, roasted meat symbolized a link between the notions of meat eating and physical strength. Montanari summarizes that there was an "inevitable equation between strength and power, and an equal link between meat and power" [13].

Although meat was emphasized in the early cultures of the Middle Ages, the Mediterranean diet researched in the Rockefeller Foundation Studies in the early 1950s showed a diet that was near vegetarian [14]. This near-vegetarian diet contained specific nutrient and non-nutrient components, antioxidant vitamins, fiber, and a variety of phenolic compounds [15–17]. Investigators in this study conducted 7-day weighed food inventories on 128 households, and 7-day dietary intake records were obtained on 7500 persons in those households. A food frequency questionnaire was administered to 765 households.

An additional study conducted by the European Atomic Energy Commission (EURATOM) compared nine regions in northern Europe and two in southern Europe (both in southern Italy) [15]. Investigators in this study conducted 7 consecutive days of dietary interviews on 3725 families and weighed all foods present in the households on those 7 days. The study showed that although there were no consistent north-south variations in overall intake of table fat, the foods that contributed fat to the diets in the two regions were different. In the northern regions butter and margarine were consumed in larger quantities. In the southern two regions margarine was not consumed at all and the principal fat was olive oil. Additionally, in the southern regions, greater amounts of cereals, vegetables, fruit, and fish were eaten with smaller intakes of potatoes, meat, dairy foods, eggs, and sweets described.

1.2 MEDITERRANEAN POPULATIONS AND THEIR CHANGING DIETARY PATTERNS

Although these studies in the 1960s indicate very healthy eating habits, studies today in Crete, where investigators used 24-hour recall data with biomarkers to assess intakes, showed a decrease in bread, fruit, potatoes, and olive oil with increases in meat, fish, and cheese [19]. These data were compared to that collected by Kromhout and his colleagues in the 1960s [20]. Italian cuisine has also followed this same path [21]. Food balance data collected in this region since the 1960s indicate that the availability of meat, dairy products, and animal fats has increased [22, 23].

A more recent study by Trichopoulou and his colleagues in Crete shows that greater adherence to the traditional Mediterranean diet results in significant decreases in overall mortality [24]. For death due to coronary heart disease and cancer, an inverse association was found in the group of persons who adhered to the diet. It is interesting to note that associations between individual food groups and total mortality did not show statistical significance.

1.3 AMERICAN CHANGES IN DIETARY PATTERNS AND ORIGINS

The Mediterranean diet has very distinct origins. Many healthy eating habits in the 1960s were a carryover from ancient times. Just as the Mediterranean diet is changing today in comparison to the 1960s, the American diet is also undergoing alterations.

Greg Critser in his book, *Fat Land*, chronicles the increase in obesity in America by describing political and food industry roles in changing the type and amount of food we eat [25]. He begins by describing the agricultural secretary's push to enlarge the farmer's marketplace and increase corn production. By the mid-1970s its production was at an all-time high leading to an equivalent increase in farmers' income. Critser describes these corn surpluses as a spur to those makers of convenience foods who now focused on new-product development and sales.

In 1971 Japanese scientists developed a cheaper sweetener called high-fructose corn syrup, HFCS [26]. Compared to cane sugar, it was six times sweeter, and because it was a corn product, the cost of production was drastically reduced. Also, its preservation properties, such as preventing freezer burn and increasing shelf-life of products made it a sought-out item.

In addition to its properties of sweetness and stability there are other characteristics of HFCS that affect our physiology. Compared to sucrose, fructose bypasses many critical intermediary paths and goes directly to the liver, where it is used as a building block for triglycerides. It then

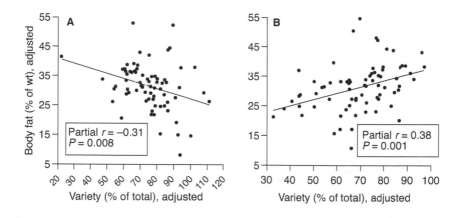

Figure 1.1 The associations between body fatness and dietary variety obtained from vegetables (A) and sweets, snacks, condiments, entrées, and carbohydrates (B). Partial correlations are shown, meaning that each relation is adjusted for age, sex, and dietary variety in the other food group. With the effects of age and sex controlled for in multiple regression analysis on percentage body fat, the variety of vegetables consumed was inversely associated with body fatness, and the variety of sweets, snacks, condiments, entrées, and carbohydrates consumed was positively associated with body fatness (overall R2 = 0.46, P < 0.0001) [31].

causes an increase in fatty acids in the blood. When muscle tissue is exposed to excessive levels of fatty acids, the result is a resistance to insulin that leads to type 2 diabetes [27, 28].

At the University of Minnesota, John Bantle, who has worked in a variety of National Institutes of Health studies, including the Diabetes Control and Complications Trial, used a clinical trial study design with two dozen healthy volunteers who consumed a diet containing 17% of their calories from fructose. Secondly, those same subjects were switched to a diet sweetened mainly with sucrose. The results of the study showed that the fructose diet produced significantly higher triglycerides than the sucrose-sweetened diet [29]. Hollenbeck further points to the negative aspects of fructose by concluding that the harmful effects of fructose appear to be greater for those at an increased coronary heart disease risk [30].

McCrory and his colleagues provide the data in Figure 1.1 and Figure 1.2 to show the connection between fructose-laden foods and BMI [31].

In the mid-1970s palm oil became the focus as a fat source similar to HFCS for sugar. Just as HFCS had very positive sweetening properties, palm oil also provided stabilizing properties to allow products to last for long periods of time on the supermarket shelves [32]. Because palm oil was from a vegetable source, few saw its highly saturated characteristics as a potential medical problem. Because of regulations around foods, their

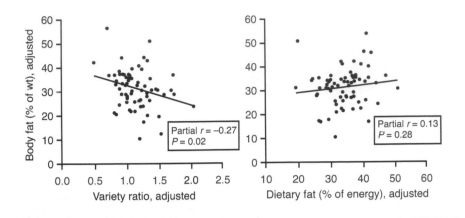

Figure 1.2 Associations between body fatness and the variety ratio, calculated as the ratio of the variety of vegetables to the variety of sweets, snacks, condiments, entrées, and carbohydrates (adjusted for age, sex, and percentage dietary fat), and percentage dietary fat (adjusted for age, sex, and the variety ratio). When the variety ratio and dietary fat were included in the same regression model, dietary fat was not significantly associated with body fatness ($R2 = 0.44$, $P < 0.0001$) [31].

long-term medical implications were not considered as important as immediate purity and ability to stabilize food products where a long shelf life was needed.

In addition to the insertion of HFCS and palm oil into our food economy, fast-food chains in the 1970s played a role in increasing the amount of foods Americans eat. Greg Critser describes the super-sizing phenomenon and how it became popular [33]. He attributes the increase in super-sizing to fast food companies' designs on increasing per product margin. The concept is that the super-sized product is one costing the company only a small amount. To super-size this type of item means that more customers spend just a little more but feel that they have purchased more for the money. This marketing strategy led to increased sales and repeat purchases. It allowed the American public to eat more without purchasing double items, resulting in feelings of gluttony.

The USDA graphically depicts the changes in our American culture that over time have contributed to increases in caloric consumption (http://public.bcm.tmc.edu/pa/iortiondist.htm). Figure 1.3 shows examples of portioning changes over time.

Critser provides a variety of reasons for why American caloric intake is out of control. He focuses first on the fact that two catalysts were responsible for what he terms "boundary-free" eating in American culture. One is individual freedom where women in the 1960s and 1970s made

Do you suffer 'Portion Distortion'?

If you think food portions are bigger than they used to be, you're right. Take a look at how "typical" restaurant portion sizes have grown over the past 20 years or so:

Food	Portion Size	
	Was	Now
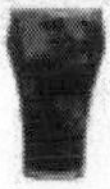 Soda	6 ounces (85 calories)	20 ounces (300 calories)
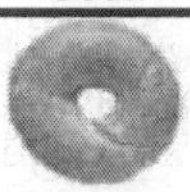 Bagel	3-inch diameter (140 calories)	5 to 6 inches (350 calories or more)
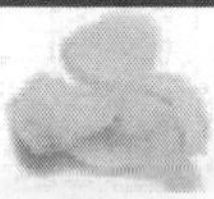 Chips	1 oz. bag (150 calories)	1.75 oz. "Grab Bag" (about 260 calories)
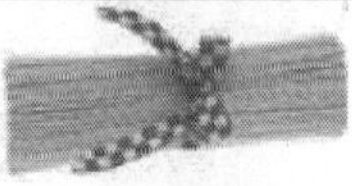 Pasta	2 cups (280 calories without sauce or fat)	4 cups or more (560 calories or more without sauce or fat)
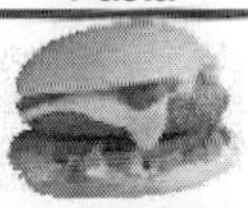 Burger	2 oz. patty + bun (270 calories)	4 oz. patty + bun (430 calories)
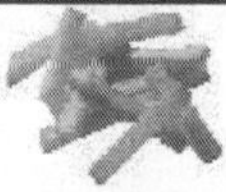 French Fries	2 ounces (210 calories)	5 ounces (540 calories)
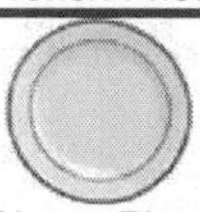 Dinner Plate	10-inch diameter	12-1/2 inch diameter

Developed by the Children's Nutrition Research Center

Before blaming your local restaurateur for your family's growing waistlines, take an honest look at how you "value" dining out experiences. According to the National Restaurant Association's Dinner Decision Making study, most consumers rank portion size as one of the 10 "hallmarks of a great place."

Figure 1.3   Examples of portioning changes over time. See http://public.bcm. tmc.edu/pa/portiondist.htm.

Table 1.3 Changes over Time in Foods Eaten Away from Home

Year	Percent of the Food Dollar Eaten Away From Home
1970	25
1985	35
1996	40

Source: Lin, B.H., Guthrie, J., Frazao, E., Nutrient contribution of foods eaten away from home, in *America's Eating Habits: Changes and Consequences*, Frazao, E., Ed., Agriculture Information Bulletin 750, USDA, Washington, DC, 1999, 213.

Table 1.4

Year	Snacks Consumed Away from Home (%)	Proportion of Meals Consumed Away from Home (%)
1977	17	16
1987	20	24
1995	22	29

Source: Lin, B.H., Guthrie, J., Frazao, E., Nutrient contribution of foods eaten away from home, in *America's Eating Habits: Changes and Consequences*, Frazao, E., Ed., Agriculture Information Bulletin 750, USDA, Washington, DC, 1999, 213.

up a large portion of the workforce. This change modified the traditional family table of the 1950s in the evenings. It now became more advantageous to eat out or order in, often not eating around a dinner table. Table 1.3 and Table 1.4 show that this change in culture was reflected in the consumption statistics of Americans. Figure 1.4 illustrates changes in daily caloric consumption in the U.S., 1910–2000.

To provide the general public with easy-to-understand concepts about healthy eating, the USDA created the Food Guide Pyramid. Figure 1.5 has a comparison of the current USDA Food Guide Pyramid and the Mediterranean Food Guide Pyramid. Also shown in that figure are two other emerging pyramids focused on food groups: The Harvard Medical School

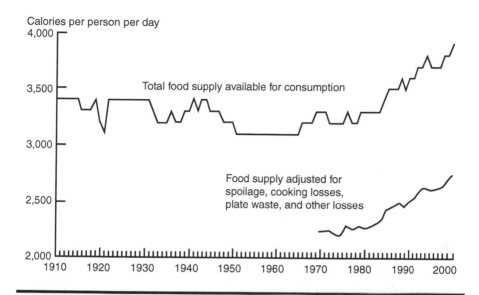

Figure 1.4   Daily calorie consumption in the U.S., 1910–2000. (Source: Putnam, J., Alishouse, J., and Kantor, L. S. 2002. U.S. per capita food supply trends: more calories, refined carbohydrates, and fats. *Food Review* 25(3):2–15.)

Guide to Healthy Eating and the Prader-Willi Syndrome Food Pyramid. Each pyramid has a different food group focus.

1.4   CONCLUSION

The concept of lifestyle change requires that we understand first where we are in terms of eating styles (American food habits) and where we might go in terms of dietary pattern (Mediterranean diet and lifestyle). This book focuses on lifestyle change and how that might be accomplished in an American culture dictated by time and efficiency. Strategies for change presented in this text were and are used in a variety of randomized controlled clinical trials where lifestyle change for extended periods of time must be maintained. Additional research on maintenance of lifestyle change is currently being studied in randomized controlled clinical trials. These trials will provide evidence of methods to help maintain lifestyle change. Examples of some of these as-yet-unstudied maintenance strategies are described in the chapters that follow.

The purpose of this text is to expose students with an interest in dietary and lifestyle change to an understanding of methods related to achieving that change. Examples of problem situations and diet change strategies will be included.

U.S.D.A. Food Guide Pyramid

Anatomy of MyPyramid

One size doesn't fit all
USDA's new MyPyramid symbolizes a personalized approach to healthy eating and physical activity. The symbol has been designed to be simple. It has been developed to remind consumers to make healthy food choices and to be active every day. The different parts of the symbol are described below.

Activity
Activity is represented by the steps and the person climbing them, as a reminder of the importance of daily physical activity.

Moderation
Moderation is represented by the narrowing of each food group from bottom to top. The wider base stands for foods with little or no solid fats or added sugars. These should be selected more often. The narrower top area stands for foods containing more added sugars and solid fats. The more active you are, the more of these foods can fit into your diet.

Personalization
Personalization is shown by the person on the steps, the slogan, and the URL. Find the kinds and amounts of food to eat each day at MyPyramid.gov.

Proportionality
Proportionality is shown by the different widths of the food group bands. The widths suggest how much food a person should choose from each group. The widths are just a general guide, not exact proportions. Check the Web site for how much is right for you.

Variety
Variety is symbolized by the 6 color bands representing the 5 food groups of the Pyramid and oils. This illustrates that foods from all groups are needed each day for good health.

Gradual Improvement
Gradual improvement is encouraged by the slogan. It suggests that individuals can benefit from taking small steps to improve their diet and lifestyle each day.

MyPyramid.gov
STEPS TO A HEALTHIER YOU

| GRAINS | VEGETABLES | FRUITS | MILK | MEAT & BEANS |

http://www.mypyramid.gov/downloads/MyPyramid_Anatomy.pdf

- Provides nutritional guidelines for Americans
- Emphasizes consumption of grain products, fruits, and vegetables
- _____

Harvard School of Public Health "Healthy Eating" Pyramid

Healthy Eating Pyramid

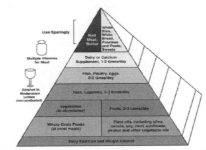

http://www.hsph.harvard.edu/nutritionsource/pyramids.html

- Emphasizes a mostly plant-based diet, including unsaturated oils
- Discourages consumption of red meat and refined carbohydrates
- Includes guidelines for exercise, weight control, alcohol intake, and supplement use

Figure 1.5   Comparison of the current USDA Food Guide Pyramid and the Mediterranean Food Guide Pyramid. Also shown are two other emerging pyramids focused on food groups: The Harvard Medical School Guide to Healthy Eating and the Prader-Willi Syndrome Food Pyramid. Each pyramid has a different food group focus.

Vegetarian Diet Pyramid

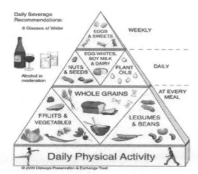

- Provides nutritional guidelines for persons following a vegetarian diet
- Emphasizes whole grains, fruits, vegetables, and legumes
- Includes alternatives to dairy products
- Discourages frequent egg consumption

http://www.oldwayspt.org/pyramids/veg/p_veg.html

Traditional Latin-American Diet

Pyramid

- Emphasizes foods specific to the traditional diets of Latin America
- Discourages egg and red meat consumption
- Includes dairy, poultry, fish, and shellfish as protein sources

http://www.oldwayspt.org/pyramids/latin/p_latin.html

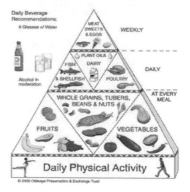

Figure 1.5 *Continued.*

Traditional Mediterranean Diet

Pyramid

- Emphasizes consumption of starchy foods
- Includes foods common to traditional Mediterranean diets
- Discourages red meat consumption
- Recommends fish, yogurt, and cheese as primary protein sources

http://www.oldwayspt.org/pyramids/med/

p_med.html

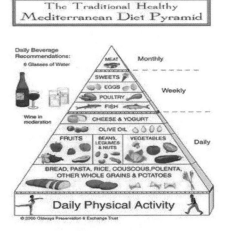

Traditional Asian Diet Pyramid

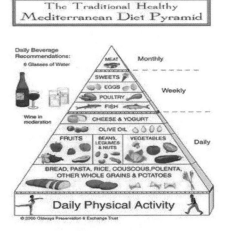

- Includes foods and beverages popular within traditional Asian diets
- Emphasizes consumption of grain products
- Recommends fish, shellfish, and dairy as main protein sources

http://www.oldwayspt.org/pyramids/asian/p_asian.html

Figure 1.5 *Continued.*

Activity Pyramid for Children

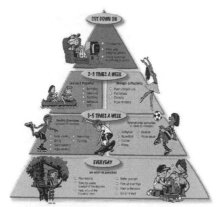

- Provides activity guidelines for children
- Includes pictures of various activities
- Emphasizes an active lifestyle
- Includes guidelines for everyday activities, sports, aerobic exercise, leisure activities, strength training, and secondary activities

http://www.classbrain.com/artread/publish/article_31.shtml

Food Pyramid for Young Children

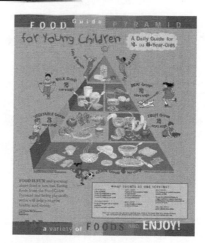

- Provides nutritional recommendations for children ages 2-6 years
- Includes serving size information
- Emphasizes variety within the diet
- Provides colorful pictures created for children

http://www.usda.gov/cnpp/KidsPyra/BIGpyr.pdf

Figure 1.5   *Continued.*

Food Pyramid for Older Adults

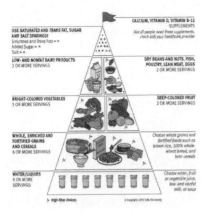

- Provides nutritional guidelines for adults aged 70 years and older
- Narrow shape of pyramid emphasizes a reduction in energy intake
- Focuses on nutrient-dense, antioxidant-rich foods
- Emphasizes adequate fluid and fiber intake

http://nutrition.tufts.edu/pdf/pyramid.pdf

Prader-Willi Syndrome Food Pyramid

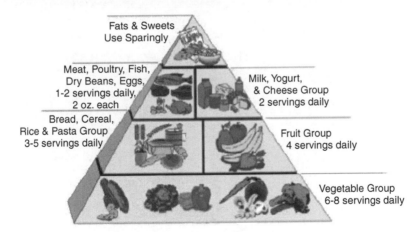

- Provides dietary recommendations for individuals with Prader-Willi Syndrome
- Emphasizes vegetable consumption to help prevent excessive energy intake
- Aims to facilitate weight control

http://www.pwsausa.org/syndrome/foodpyramid.htm

Figure 1.5 *Continued.*

REFERENCES

1. Nestle, M., Mediterranean diets: historical and research overview, *Am. J. Nutr.,* 61(Suppl), 1313S, 1995.
2. World Health Organization, *World Health Statistics Annual,* 1993, Geneva, 1994.
3. Keys, A., Coronary heart disease in seven countries, *Circulation,* 41, 1, 1970.
4. Gussou, J.D. and Akabas, S., Are we really fixing up the food supply?, *J. Am. Diet. Assoc.,* 93, 1300, 1993.
5. Nestle, M., Traditional models of healthy eating: alternatives to "techno-food," *J. Nutr. Educ.,* 26, 241, 1994.
6. Darby, W.J., Ghalioungui, P., and Grivetti, L., *Food: The Gift of Osiris,* Vols 1 and 2, London: Academic Press, 1997.
7. Vermeule, E., *Greece in the Bronze Age,* Chicago: University of Chicago Press, 1964.
8. Vickery, K.F., Food in early Greece, *Illinois Studies Social Sciences,* 20, 1, 1936.
9. Seymour, T.D., *Life in the Homeric Age,* New York: The Macmillan Co., 1907, 208.
10. Yonge, C., *The Deipnosophists or Banquet of the Learned of Athens,* Vols 1–3, London: George Bell and Sons, 1907.
11. Montanari, M., Romans, barbarians, Christians: the dawn of European food culture, in *Food: A Culinary History,* Flandrin, J.-L. and Montanari, M., Eds., New York: Columbia United Press, 1999, 165.
12. Montanari, M., Production structures and food systems in the early Middle Ages, in *Food: A Culinary History,* Flandrin, J. and Montanari, M., Eds., New York: Columbia United Press, 1999, 168.
13. Montanari, M., Peasants, warriors, priests: images of society styles of diet, in *Food: A Culinary History,* Flandrin, J. and Montanari, M., Eds., New York: Columbia United Press, 1999, 178.
14. Allbaugh, L.G., Crete: a case study of an underdeveloped area, Princeton, NJ: Princeton University Press, 1953.
15. Dwyer, J.T., Vegetarian eating patterns: science, values and food choices — where do we go from here? *Am. J. Clin. Nut.,* 59, 1255S, 1994.
16. Kashi, L.E., Lenart, E.B., and Willett, W.C., Health implications of Mediterranean diets in the light of contemporary knowledge. I. Plant foods and dairy products. *Am. J. Clin. Nutr.,* 61, 1407S, 1995.
17. Kushi, L.E., Lenart, E.B., and Willett, W.C., Health implications of Mediterranean diets in the light of contemporary knowledge. II. Meat, wine, fats and oils, *Am. J. Clin. Nutr.,* 61, 1416S, 1995.
18. Ferro-Luzzi, A. and Branca, F., The Mediterranean diet, Italian style: prototype of a health diet, *Am. J. Clin. Nutr.,* 61, 1338S, 1995.
19. Kafatos, A., Kouroumalis, I., Vlachonikolis, I., Theodorou, C., and Latadarios, D., Coronary heart-disease risk-factor status of the Cretan urban population in the 1980s, *Am. J. Clin. Nutr.,* 54, 591, 1991.
20. Kromhout, D., Keep, A., Aravanis, C. et al., Food consumption patterns in the 1960s in seven countries, *Am. J. Clin. Nutri.,* 49, 889, 1989.
21. Key, A., The Mediterranean diet and public health: personal reflections, *Am. J. Clin. Nutr.,* 61, 1321S, 1995.
22. Food and Agriculture Organization, Food balance sheets, 1984–1986, average, Rome: Food and Agriculture Organization, 1991.

23. Serra-Majem, L. and Helsing, E., Changing patterns of fat in Mediterranean countries, *Eur. J. Clin. Nutr., 47,* 1993.
24. Trichopoulou, A., Costacou, T., Bamia, C., and Trichopoulos, D., Adherence to a Mediterranean diet and survival in a Greek population, *N. Engl. J. Med.,* 348, 2599, 2003.
25. Critser, G., *Fat Land*, Boston: Houghton Mifflin Company, 2003, 7 [or Chapter 1].
26. Hanover, L.M. and White, J.S., Manufacturing, composition and applications of fructose, *Am. J. Clin. Nutr.,* 58, 724 S, 1993.
27. Vines, G., Sweet but deadly, *New Scientist,* 26, September 1, 2001.
28. Thorburn, A.W. and Storlein, L.H. et al., Fructose-induced in vivo insulin resistance and elevated plasma triglyceride levels in rats, *Am. J. Clin. Nutr.,* 49, 1155, 1989.
29. Bantle, J.P. and Raatz, S.K. et al., Effects of dietary fructose on plasma lipids in healthy subjects, *Am. J. Clin. Nutr.,* 72, 1128, 2000.
30. Hollenbeck, C.B., Dietary fructose effects on lipoprotein metabolism and risk for coronary artery disease, *Am. J. Clin. Nutr.,* 58, s800, 1993.
31. McCrory, M.A. and Fuss, P.J. et al., Dietary variety within food groups: association with energy intake and body fatness in men and women, *Am. J. Clin. Nutr.,* 69, 440, 1999.
32. Pletcher, J., Regulation with growth: the political economy of palm oil in Malaysia, *World Development,* 19, 623, 1991.
33. Critser, G., *Fat Land*, Boston: Houghton Mifflin Company, 2003, 20 [or Chapter 2].

2

ASSESSMENT OF LIFE CYCLE FACTORS RELATED TO DIET AND OBESITY-ASSOCIATED DISEASE

2.1 PREVENTION IN CHILDHOOD: STAGE 1

The childhood obesity epidemic is the critical health issue of our time. Researchers express concern that being overweight or obese in childhood will lead to health-related problems in adulthood. Indeed studies show that atherosclerosis begins in childhood and progresses into adulthood, leading to coronary heart disease (CHD) [1]. Childhood obesity is associated with increases in coronary artery fibrous plaques later in life [2]. Some of the strongest evidence of the relationship between obesity in childhood and disease comes from an analysis of the long-term follow-up of the Harvard Growth Study [3]. This study found 55 years after participation that obesity in adolescence increased the risk of disease and death regardless of subsequent adult body composition for men. The relative risk for all-cause mortality was 2.3, and 1.8 for coronary heart disease, in adults who were overweight as youth compared to adults who were lean as youth. Steinberger et al. reported that BMI at age 13 was correlated highly with BMI and total LDL cholesterol at age 22, and inversely correlated with glucose utilization [4]. The Bogalusa Heart Study confirmed that clustering of risk factors in childhood tracks into adulthood [5].

There is strong evidence that diets high in vegetables and fruits, with consumption above the National Cancer Institute recommendations of five servings each day, protect against the development of cancers at many sites [6–16]. Childhood eating excesses are precursors for cancer and track into adulthood [6–16].

It is clear that significant health risks related to obesity exist during childhood as well. Obesity early in life is associated with hypertension (systolic and diastolic blood pressure), hypercholesterolemia, hypertri-glyceridemia, increased low-density lipoprotcins, decreased high-density lipoproteins, and impaired glucose tolerance [17–19, 20a,b, 21]. In one study researchers used ultrasound to look at the arteries of 48 severely obese children compared to children of normal weight [22]. The obese children showed signs of poor artery health, including stiffness in the artery walls and general decline in artery lining function.

2.1.1 Eating Habits of Children and Adolescents in Relation to the Dietary Guidelines

In 1999 only 23.9% of adolescents had eaten the Dietary Guidelines recommendation of five or more servings of fruits or vegetables a day during the previous week [23]. Jahns et al. report on a nationally representative study of children ages 2 to 18 years conducted in 1977 to 1978, 1989 to 1991, and 1994 to 1996. For all age groups the percentage of children who snack between meals increased from 77% to 91% [24], and the average number of snacks per day increased by 24%, with the average daily calorie intake from snacking increasing by 30%.

2.1.2 Fostering Patterns of Preference Consistent with Healthier Diets in the Very Young

Data indicate that food preferences are learned based on experience with food and eating [25, 26]. Skinner and colleagues showed in a longitudinal study that food preferences are set by the age of 3 to 4 years [27]. The data suggest that the best chance to foster patterns of preference consistent with healthier diets might be to focus on the very young [27, 28].

Depending on the foods that are available, children's learned food preferences can either promote or impede the consumption of nutritionally adequate diets. The availability of large portions of energy-dense foods, high in sugar, fat, and salt contributes to an environment that is conducive to obesity [20a,b]. Studies show that genetic predispositions bias us to like sweet and salty foods that are more energy dense over the energy dilute [29–32]. New foods that are not sweet or salty, for example healthy foods such as vegetables, will initially be rejected. Fortunately children learn to like many foods if allowed to begin eating them early in life when eating patterns are just beginning to form [29].

Food neophobia, or fear of the new, is manifested in avoidance of new foods. The timing of weaning and introduction of solid foods varies with different cultures. Nutrition guidance in the U.S. is that by the second half of the first year (6 months), an exclusive breast milk or formula diet does not provide adequate nutrition, and the introduction of solid foods is recommended [33, 34]. Recent advice indicates the age of 4 to 6 months for beginning solids, and that very few infants will need anything other than breast milk or an infant formula before 4 months, and almost all infants will need extra solid foods after the age of 6 months [35]. It is at this point in development that the predisposition to respond neophobically to new foods begins to influence food preferences and intake. Research shows that children's food preferences are strongly correlated with food consumption. Domel reports that, among infants just beginning the transition to solid foods, the neophobic response appears to be minimal [48].In this research mothers introduced 4- to 6-month-old infants to new fruits or vegetables by feeding one new food to the infant over a series of 10 lunches. Results indicated that only one feeding of a new food increased the mean intake of 30 grams at the first feeding to a mean of 60 grams at the second feeding. Additionally, if an infant had experience with one vegetable, other vegetables were more readily eaten. This is in contrast to patterns seen in toddlers, preschool children, and adults, where numerous exposures to a food are needed to set a preference for that food. Birch's research shows that by the time children reach 2 to 5 years of age, approximately 5 to 10 exposures to a new food are needed to produce significant increases in children's preferences. Minimal neophobia might be adaptive during infancy, a period when primarily adults control access to food and infants are not mobile enough to select food for themselves [37]. Neophobia is minimal in infancy, increases through early childhood, and declines from early childhood to adulthood [38–43]. Recently, Skinner and colleagues showed in a longitudinal study that the strongest predictors of the number of foods liked at 8 years of age were the number of foods liked at 4 years and the food neophobia score [27].

2.1.3 Parental Influences on Children's Food Preferences and Patterns

Three parental factors influence children's food preferences and patterns: the foods they make available to the child, the types of child feeding practices they use, and their own eating behavior [44].

2.1.3.1 Availability of Foods

Researchers show that when the environment provides nutrient-dense and calorie-sparse foods (fruits and vegetables) children consume more of them [45–48]. Age plays a role in the acceptance of foods available to children. As described in more detail above, Birch et al. found that 4- to 7-month-old infants need minimal experience with a new food in order to prefer it [36] and, additionally, that this new food enhances the infants' acceptance of other similar foods. This is in contrast to findings noted in 2- to 5-year-old children who seem to need multiple exposures to a new food before significant increases in intake are noted [49–51]. Data from the Framingham Children's Study suggest that dietary behaviors related to CVD aggregate within families, thus illustrating the connection between availability of food and eventual disease [52].

2.1.3.2 Types of Child Feeding Practices

Fisher and Birch studied the negative effects of restricting access to foods [53, 54]. In girls, high levels of restricting access resulted in higher levels of snack food intake. Higher levels of adiposity in both boys and girls predicted higher levels of maternal restriction [53]. In another study, restricting access to palatable foods resulted in increasing both boys' and girls' selection of that food within the restricted context. Those researchers also showed that the child's weight status was positively related to parental restriction with higher levels of reported restriction associated with higher relative weight (weight for height) in children [54].

Studies show a negative association comparing parents' use of pressure and girls' fruit and vegetable intake [37, 55]. Specifically, pressure in child feeding might have negative influences on children's eating that extends beyond preferences for particular foods [56–58] or foods eaten at specific meals [59] to include more broad characteristics of children's diets like fruit and vegetable intake. Parent–child interactions involving vegetables eaten at dinner are important because a young child considers vegetables a "meal" food [60]. Baranowski and his colleagues present data showing that a sizeable portion of school-age children's fruit and vegetable intake occurs at dinner [61]. Parents' "do as I say" pressure on children to finish their vegetables during a meal is one way of encouraging children to eat. Research shows that offering food to obtain a reward decreases prefer-ences for that food [56–58]. Very importantly, two studies show that pressuring children to eat may diminish their ability to self-regulate intake based on appetite. In a recent study, mothers with higher concerns about the role of fruit and vegetable intake in preventing disease had children who consumed fewer servings of vegetables [62]. Although those research-ers did not measure child-feeding practices, their data suggest that mothers who reported greater concern about the role of fruit and vegetables in disease prevention might have applied more pressure to their children to eat vegetables. These data point to the importance of additional research to investigate the influence of parents' feeding practices on children's fruit and vegetable intake.

Fisher researched this important question by evaluating parents' use of pressure to eat as predictors of their 5-year-old daughters' fruit and vegetable, macronutrient, and fat intakes. The study showed that pressure to eat fruits and vegetables resulted in daughters who consumed fewer servings of fruits and vegetables [44].

Dr. Leann Birch developed the Child Feeding Questionnaire (CFQ) to provide information on how restrictive or unrestrictive parents are in terms of child-feeding practices [63]. Research is needed to assess the effect of feeding practices on populations of ethnicity and disadvantaged groups. Some preliminary research shows that, in populations where the ability to purchase food is compromised, often lack of structure and restriction related to feeding practices is common [64, 65]. Often in these groups, poor eating practices in childhood are due to a lack of parental guidance and modeling.

2.1.3.3 Parental Modeling of Eating Behavior

Limited data show that modeling can be effective in inducing children to like new foods [66] or foods they previously disliked [67, 68]. Studies suggest that strong modeling influences occur in the context of the following factors: *observational learning* (a focus in our education intervention) when young children learn what and how to eat by watching their parents' intake and reactions to foods, thus leading children to adopt their parents' behaviors and *response facilitation* when an occurrence of an eating behavior is frequent and interactive. (Children who help their mothers pick and eat cherry tomatoes out of the garden might request to eat their own tomato.) [28, 66, 67, 69–72].

2.1.4 Parental Eating Habits Mirror Those in Their Young Children

Pliner and Pelchat tabulated the likes and dislikes of target children and their parents. The results revealed that study children resembled their parents in their food preferences [73]. Oliveria and her colleagues confirmed a statistically significant but modest correlation ($r < 0.50$) found between parents and children's intakes for most nutrients [52]. This Framingham Children's Study also demonstrated that parents' eating patterns have a significant relationship to the nutrient intake of their preschool children, particularly with regards to saturated fat, total fat, and cholesterol. Other researchers examining familial aggregation of nutrient intake between parents and their children have found similarities in nutrient intake [26, 67, 74–76].

2.1.5 Existing Family-Based Interventions

Parents and caregivers have an important and lasting influence on the eating habits of school-age children. Studies of children ages 6 to 11 years, where parents were targeted as the primary mediators of change, showed greater weight loss, increased number of behavioral changes, and better retention in the study [77, 78]. A randomized community trial in St. Paul, Minnesota, showed that multicomponent school-based programs can increase fruit and vegetable consumption among children in the 4th and 5th grades [79]. One aspect of the study involved the "home team" approach, where parents and children participated in activities brought home by the student. Epstein and coworkers used a prospective, randomized, controlled design to examine the effects of behavioral family-based treatment on percent overweight and growth over 10 years in obese 6- to 12-year-old children [80]. Obese children and their parents were randomized to three groups that were provided similar diet, exercise, and behavior management training but differed in the reinforcement for weight loss and behavior change. The child and parent group reinforced parent and child behavior change and weight loss, the child group reinforced child behavior change and weight loss, and the nonspecific control group reinforced families for attendance. Children in the child and parent group showed significantly greater decreases in percent overweight after 5 and 10 years than children in the nonspecific control group. Children in the child group showed increases in percent overweight after 5 and 10 years that were midway between the child and parent and nonspecific groups — and not significantly different from either.

To this author's knowledge there is no existing work in very young children just beginning to form eating habits where strategies are taught to parents to change their existing feeding practices. A few programs are in progress where older preschool children are involved along with family members with the goal of change in both children and parents. For children, the parent is the primary mediator of change, and a family-based intervention is appropriate [81].

In an ongoing study, preschool children are targeted in Head Start centers in the New York area to reduce cardiovascular risk factors. Specific aims include reducing blood cholesterol, reducing dietary intake of total and saturated fat in school meals, and increasing nutrition knowledge among the 3-year-old children involved in this study for the next 3 years [82].

The Parent As Teachers (PAT) program is a national parent education project for underserved populations that focuses on promoting positive childrearing practices, but it does not include a diet component. In the state of Missouri, researchers have combined PAT with the High 5, Low Fat Program (H5LF) focusing on teaching African-American parents to be good models of behavior with an emphasis on fruit and vegetable intake. Preliminary results show modest increases in fruit and vegetable intake in parents of children where modeling of healthy eating behaviors occurs [83].

St. Jeor describes a study that is in pilot stages for preschool children, Health Opportunities for Pre-School Children to Optimize Their Cardiovascular Health (HOPSCOTCH) [81]. The purpose of this study is to develop and test the feasibility of a family-based, weight management program. Overweight parents with their preschool children who have already established many eating habits that might result in patterns contrary to the USDA Dietary Guidelines were enrolled. As pairs they were randomized into either a treatment group, with the parent as the mediator of change, or a control group. The child intervention provides age-specific, healthy eating patterns with increases in daily physical activity in order to enable weight stabilization or small weight gains of not more than 2 kg (4 to 5 lb) per year. This will allow for gradual declines in BMI as the child grows. The intervention for the parent (mother as the major caregiver) traditionally emphasizes a weight loss of 500 kcal/day (1 lb/wk) and prevention of weight regain. The parent-and-child pairs attend all sessions together. After a brief socialization activity, the children are taken to a play/educational group while the parents attend group treatment sessions. The session ends with the parent-and-child groups combined, and the children help the parent prepare a snack. Data is not yet available to indicate study results.

2.2 REMEDIATION IN CHILDREN AND ADOLESCENTS: STAGE 2

2.2.1 Family-Based Interventions in Older Children

Diet Intervention Study in Children (DISC): In this study we counseled parents of children whose serum cholesterol was found to be above normal. We focused on decreasing saturated fat and increasing fruits and vegetables in 7- to 10-year-old children's diets, with intervention follow-up through age 18. After 3 years the statistically significant data showed that the children in this study lowered their LDL cholesterol levels by following a fat-modified diet that also focused on consumption of fruits and vegetables [84].

Following year 3 in DISC, we used motivational interviewing techniques to intensify our intervention with study subjects who had reached their teens. Also at this time we counseled parents using an educational intervention. We emphasized their interactions with their teenagers regarding the ways they dealt with their teen's poor eating habits at times when life was rushed and stressful [85].

Study of Nutrition in Teens (SONIT): In this study we worked intensively with parents of children whose LDL cholesterol was above the 50th percentile. Our team of nutritionists developed interventions and corresponding materials focused on changing adolescents' eating habits to make them lower in saturated fat with an increase in fruits and vegetables. Data from this study showed changes in teen eating habits following educational sessions with them and their parents. Motivational interviewing techniques were used when eating habits did not conform to study goals for saturated fat and fruit and vegetable intake [86].

Trial of Ready-to-Eat Cereal (TREC): This study looked at changes in serum cholesterol in children and parents following a feeding study where cereal was supplied to families. One cereal product was high in folate, and the other was not. Both cereals looked identical. Our team of nutritionists developed materials to implement behavior-change strategies focused on facilitating change in parents and children to decrease saturated fat and increase fruits and vegetables.

Diabetes Control and Complications Trial (DCCT): In this study we emphasized a diet low in saturated fat and high in fruits and vegetables. Clinically this study showed the importance of parental influences on children with diabetes. Often we counseled adolescents with eating disorders who described intense parental control over their childhood eating behaviors. Well-meaning parents often used very restrictive eating practices to achieve the greatest decrease in blood glucose levels. The result was an adult dealing with diabetes with very unhealthy eating behaviors [87, 88].

2.3   REMEDIATION IN ADULTS: STAGE 3

Lipid Research Clinic Studies: The Lipid Research Clinic Studies were designed to change the level of dietary fat and cholesterol in diets of men who were also taking a cholesterol drug [89, 90]. We currently counsel Lipid Research Study participants in a variety of clinical studies to adhere to the National Cholesterol Education Program (NCEP) Step 1 and 2 nutrition recommendations.

Modification of Diet in Renal Disease Study (MDRD): In this study nutrition lifestyle change was used to try to delay progression to dialysis in patients with diagnosed renal disease. Nutrition counselors implemented a complex diet requiring expert skill in compliance monitoring and strategies to enhance dietary adherence. The diet in this study was modified in protein and phosphorus [91].

Adherence to a very difficult dietary pattern was based on self-management skills and included simplistic messages relative to negotiated action plans [92]. With many nutrients to assess and then modify for optimum laboratory parameters in patients, we simplified by asking the patient to focus on one main nutrient, protein, while the nutrition interventionist selected a food contributing high levels of another nutrient in need of modification, such as potassium, and demonstrated how to reduce that one food to lower potassium intake. The patient made decisions about what foods to change to modify protein. This meant selecting foods that were most easily reduced in quantity, and changing portions. Often a substitute for the food high in protein designed to reduce protein intake was chosen by the patient. Because protein reduction requires an increase in caloric consumption to reduce the possibility of muscle wasting, patients selected foods that contributed calories without adding large amounts of protein to the diet.

Women's Health Initiative (WHI): In this study lasting for 10 years, postmenopausal women were asked to follow a low-fat eating pattern with increased fruits, vegetables, and grains. A substudy was completed using motivational interviewing [93].

Elderly women in this study participated in groups designed to facilitate dietary fat reduction and increase fruit and vegetable and grain servings. Motivational interviewing changed the adherence levels in participants in the study by asking each participant to look at graphs of their dietary compliance over time and evaluate that graph providing insight into why adherence to dietary prescription might have fallen over time. For women who were having difficulty with dietary adherence, this process provided a recheck of what lifestyle changes might have caused lapses in diet adherence.

Lifestyle change in women in the WHI showed that over 7.5 years, when women in the intervention group were compared to those in the control group, two observations were demonstrated [95]. First, women in the intervention group lost weight in the first year (2.2 kg, p <.001). Those same women in the intervention group, when compared to the control group, were able to maintain that weight loss after 7.5 years (1.9 kg, p <.001 at 1 year and 0.4 kg, p =.01 at 7.5 years) [94].

In the WHI, little time was spent with the more novel approaches such as those indicated in Chapter 13, where focus is placed on feelings. In the elderly it became very evident that lifestyle changes were enormous, ranging from the loss of a spouse, children returning home after a divorce, illnesses, retirement, the deaths of friends and relatives, divorces, etc. Given the enormity of lifestyle change in the elderly and the increase in lifespan with our current generation, facilitating skills in tagging feelings is extremely important in this population.

As I remember talking with my wonderful WHI study participants, the idea of tagging feelings was not addressed to the degree that it should have been to achieve optimum dietary adherence. Poor dietary adherence was often dismissed as "life is stressful." Using ideas from Chapter 13, I might have asked each woman to go beyond this dismissal of feelings to actually tagging what feelings make dietary changes difficult.

Instead of saying "I am just too stressed to follow my eating pattern," the participant might have looked inward to feelings. "I am angry and sad that two of my best friends just died, and my husband is in the hospital. What difference does it make that I eat healthy foods? I need comfort food that is high in fat. I think I will go buy a Rueben sandwich at the deli." Instead, with skills in appropriately coping with the feelings of sadness and anger, she might have thought, "It is okay to feel sad and angry. My response to this should be crying, not eating."

Women's Intervention Nutrition Study (WINS): In this secondary prevention study, women who have had breast cancer were randomly placed on a low-fat dietary pattern or a control ad lib diet [95]. A dietary intervention was used to determine if recurrence of cancer could be prevented using nutrition lifestyle change. Motivational interviewing skills are used to counsel participants to achieve and maintain a very low-saturated fat diet with increased fruit and vegetable intake.

Once again, a focus on tagging feelings would have improved dietary adherence. In this group of women, the struggle was the emotion of fear of cancer recurrence.

The studies above show work with three stages of the lifecycle — one that involved changes in toddlers, children, and adolescents, adults and the elderly. Chapter 4 provides more detail for each of these lifecycle stages.

REFERENCES

1. PDAY Research Group, Relationship of atherosclerosis in young men to serum lipoprotein cholesterol concentrations and smoking. A preliminary report from the Pathobiological Determinants of Atherosclerosis in Youth (PDAY) Research Group, *JAMA*, 264, 3018, 1990.
2. Freedman, D.S. et al., The relation of overweight to cardiovascular risk factors among children and adolescents: The Bogalusa Heart Study, *Pediatrics*, 103, 1175, 1999.
3. Must, A. et al., Long-term morbidity and mortality of overweight adolescents, a follow-up of the Harvard Growth Study of 1922 to 1935, *N. Engl. J. Med.*, 327, 1350, 1992.
4. Steinberger, J. et al., Adiposity in childhood predicts obesity and insulin resistance and insulin resistance in young adulthood, *J. Pediatr.*, 138, 469, 2001.
5. Bao, W. et al., Persistence of multiple cardiovascular risk clustering related to Syndrome X from childhood to early adulthood: the Bogalusa Heart Study, *Arch. Intern. Med.*, 154, 1842, 1994.

6. Potter, J.D., *Food, Nutrition, and the Prevention of Cancer: A Global Perspective,* Washington, DC: American Institute for Cancer Research, 1997.
7. Reynolds, K.D. et al., Design of 'high 5': fruit and vegetable consumption for reduction of cancer risk, *J. Cancer Educ.,* 13, 169, 1998.
8. Reynolds, K.D. et al., Patterns in child and adolescent consumption of fruit and vegetables: effects of gender and ethnicity across four sites, *J. Am. Coll. Nutr.,* 18, 248, 1999.
9. Riddoch, C.J. and Boreham, C.A.G., The health-related physical activity of children, *Sports Medicine,* 19, 86, 1995.
10. Nicklas, T.A. et al., School-based programs for health-risk reduction, *Ann. N.Y. Acad. Sci.,* 208, 1997.
11. Lillie-Blanton, M. et al., Racial differences in health: Not just black and white, but shades of gray, *Annu. Rev. Public Health,* 17, 411, 1996.
12. Kimm, S.Y., The role of dietary fiber in the development and treatment of childhood obesity, *Pediatrics,* 4005, 1010, 1995.
13. Kimm, S. et al., Dietary patterns of U.S. children: implications for disease prevention, *Prev. Med.,* 19, 432, 1990.
14. Havas, S. et al., Factors associated with fruit and vegetable consumption among women participation in WIC, *J. Am. Diet. Assoc.,* 98, 1141, 1998.
15. Havas, S. et al., Five a day for better health —nine community research projects to increase fruit and vegetable consumption, *Public Health Rep.,* 110, 68, 1995.
16. McGinnis, J.M. and Foege, W.H., Actual causes of death in the United States, *JAMA,* 270, 2207, 1993.
17. Dietz, W.H. and Robinson, T.N., Assessment and treatment of childhood obesity, *Pediatr. Rev.,* 14, 337, 1993.
18. Dietz, W.H., Health consequences of obesity in youth: childhood predictors of adult obesity, *Pediatrics,* 101, 518, 1998.
19. He, Q. et al., Blood pressure is associated with body mass index in both normal and obese children, *Hypertension,* 36, 165, 2000.
20a. Hill, J.O. and Peters, J.C., Environmental contributions to the obesity epidemic, *Science,* 208, 1371, 1998.
20b. Hill, J.O. and Trowbridge, F.L., Childhood obesity: future directions and research priorities, *Pediatrics,* 101, 570, 1998.
21. Wattingney, W.A. et al., Increasing impact of obesity on serum lipids and lipoproteins in young adults. The Bogalusa Heart Study, *Arch. Intern. Med.,* 151, 2017, 1991.
22. Tounian, P. et al., Presence of increased stiffness of the common carotid artery and endothelial dysfunction in severely obese children: a prospective study, *Lancet,* 358, 1400, 2001.
23. Centers for Disease Control and Prevention, Youth Risk Behavior Surveillance–United States, 1999, *MMWR,* 49, SS, 2000.
24. Jahns, L., Siega-Riz, A.M., and Popkin, B.M., The increasing prevalence of snacking among US children from 1977 to 1996, *J. Pediatr.,* 138, 493, 2001.
25. Reed, D.R. et al., Heritable variation in food preferences and their contribution to obesity, *Behav. Genet.,* 27, 373, 1997.
26. Perusse, L. and Bouchard, C., Genetics of energy intake and food preferences, In *The Genetics of Obesity,* C. Bouchard, Ed., Boca Raton, FL: CRC Press, 1994.

27. Skinner, J. et al., Children's food preferences: a longitudinal analysis, *J. Am. Diet. Assoc.*, 102, 1638, 2002.
28. Birch, L.L., Development of food preferences, *Annu. Rev. Nutr.*, 19, 41, 1999.
29. Birch, L.L., Children's preferences for high-fat foods, *Nutr. Rev.*, 50, 249, 1992.
30. Birch, L.L. et al., Conditioned flavor preferences in young children, *Physiol. Behav.*, 47, 501, 1990.
31. Johnson, S.L., McPhee, L., and Birch, L.L., Conditioned preferences: young children prefer flavors associated with high dietary fat, *Physiol. Behav.*, 50, 1245, 1991.
32. Kern, D.L. et al., The post-ingestive consequences of fat condition preferences for flavor associated with high dietary fat, *Physiol. Behav.*, 54, 71, 1993.
33. American Academy of Pediatrics Committee on Nutrition, *Pediatric Nutrition Handbook*, 2nd ed., Elk Grove, IL: American Academy of Pediatrics, 1985.
34. Harris, G. and Booth, D.A., Infants' preferences for salt in food: its dependence upon recent dietary experience, *J. Reprod. Infant Psychol.*, 5, 97, 1987.
35. Wharton, B., Weaning: pathophysiology, practice, and policy, in *Nutrition in Pediatrics: Basic Science and Clinical Applications*, 2nd ed., Walker, W.A. and Watkins, J.B., Eds., Hamilton, B.C.: Decker, 428, 1997.
36. Birch, L.L. and Fisher, J.O., Development of eating behaviors among children and adolescents, *Pediatrics*, 101, 539, suppl, 1998b.
37. Birch, L.L., Development of food acceptance patterns in the first year of life. *Proc. Nutr. Soc.*, 57, 617, 1998.
38. Pelchat, M.L. and Pliner, P., 'Try it. You'll like it.' Effects of information on willingness to try novel foods, *Appetite*, 24, 153, 1995.
39. Pliner, P., Family resemblance in food preferences, *J. Nutr. Educ.*, 15, 137, 1983.
40. Pliner, P., Development of measures of food neophobia in children, *Appetite*, 23, 147, 1994.
41. Pliner, P. and Loewen, E.R., Temperament and food neophobia in children, *Appetite*, 28, 239, 1997.
42. McFarlane, T. and Pliner, P., Increasing willingness to taste novel foods: effects of nutrition and taste information, *Appetite*, 28, 227, 1997.
43. Koivisto, U.K. and Sjoden, P.O., Food and general neophobia in Swedish families: parent-child comparisons and relationships with serving specific foods, *Appetite*, 26, 107, 1996.
44. Fisher, J.O. et al., Parental influences on young girls' fruit and vegetable, micronutrient and fat intakes, *Am. J. Clin. Nutr.*, 102, 58, 2002.
45. Resnicow, K. et al., Social-cognitive predictors of fruit and vegetable intake in children, *Health Psychol.*, 16, 272, 1997.
46. Domel, S.B. et al., Psychosocial predictors of fruit and vegetable consumption among elementary school children, *Health Educ. Res.*, 11, 299, 1996.
47. Baranowski, T. et al., Increasing fruit and vegetable consumption among 4th and 5th grade students: results from focus groups using reciprocal determinism, *J. Nutr. Educ.*, 25, 114, 1993.
48. Domel, S.B. et al., A measure of outcome expectations for fruit and vegetable preferences among fourth and fifth grade children: Reliability and validity, *Health Education Research, Theory, and Practice*, 10, 65, 1995.
49. Birch, L.L. et al., 'Clean up your plate': effects of child feeding practices on the conditioning of meal size, *Learn Motiv.*, 301, 1987.

50. Birch, L.L. and Marlin, D.W., I don't like it; I never tried it: effects of exposure to food on two-year-old children's food preferences, *Appetite*, 4, 353, 1982.

51. Sullivan, S.A. and Birch, L.L., Pass the sugar, pass the salt: experience dictates preference, *Dev. Psychol.*, 26, 546, 1990.

52. Oliveria, S.A. et al., Parent-child relationships in nutrient intake: the Framingham Children's Study, *Am. J. Clin. Nutr.*, 56, 593, 1992.

53. Fisher, J.O. and Birch, L.L., Restricting access to foods and children's eating, *Appetite*, 32, 405, 1999a.

54. Fisher, J.O. and Birch, L.L., Restricting access to palatable foods affects children's behavioral response, food selection, and intake, *Am. J. Clin. Nutr.*, 69, 1264, 1999b.

55. Fisher, J.O. and Birch, L.L., Parents' restrictive feeding practices are associated with young girls' negative self-evaluation about eating, *J. Am. Diet. Assoc.*, 100, 1341, 2000.

56. Newman, J. and Taylor, A., Effect of a means end contingency on young children's food preferences, *J. Exp. Child Psychol.*, 200, 1992.

57. Birch, L.L. et al., Effects of instrumental consumption on children's food preference, *Appetite*, 3, 125, 1982.

58. Birch, L.L., Marlin, D.W., and Rotter, J., Eating as the 'means' activity in a contingency: effects on young children's food preference, *Child Dev.*, 55, 431, 1984.

59. Birch, L.L., The acquisition of food acceptance patterns in children, in *Eating Habits: Food, Physiology and Learned Behavior*, Boakes, R.A. and Popplewell, D.A., Eds., Chichester, England: John Wiley & Sons, 1987.

60. Kirby, S.D. et al., Children's fruit and vegetable intake: socioeconomic, adult-child regional, and urban-rural influences, *J. Nutr. Educ.*, 27, 261, 1995.

61. Baranowski, T. et al., Patterns in children's fruit and vegetable consumption by meal and day of the week, *J. Am. Coll. Nutr.*, 3, 216, 1997.

62. Gibson, E.L., Wardle, J., and Watts, C.J., Fruit and vegetable consumption, nutritional knowledge and beliefs in mothers and children, *Appetite*, 31, 205, 1998.

63. Birch, L.L., Fisher, J.O., Grimm-Thomas, K., Markey, C.N., Sawyer, R., and Johnson, S.L., Confirmatory factor analysis of the Child Feeding Questionnaire: a measure of parental attitude, beliefs and practices about child feeding and obesity proneness, *Appetite*, 36, 201, 2001.

64. Baughcum, A.E. et al., Maternal feeding practices and beliefs and their relationships to overweight in early childhood, *J. Dev. Behav. Pediatr.*, 22, 391, 2001.

65. Melgar-Quiñonez, H. and Kaiser, L., Relationship of child-feeding practices to overweight to low-income Mexican-American preschool-aged children, *J. Am. Diet. Assoc.*, 104, 110, 2004.

66. Harper, L.V. and Sanders, K.M., The effect of adults' eating on young children's acceptance of unfamiliar foods, *J. Exp. Child Psychol.*, 5, 97, 1987.

67. Birch, L.L., Effects of peer models' food choices and eating behaviors on preschoolers' food preferences, *Child Dev.*, 51, 489, 1980.

68. Duncker, K., Experimental modification of children's food preferences through social suggestion, *J. Abnormal Psychol.*, 33, 489, 1938.

69. Sallis, J.F. and Nader, P.R., Family determinants of health behavior, in *Health Behavior: Emerging Research Perspectives*, Gochman, D.S., Ed. New York: Plenum, 1998.

70. Kagan, J., The role of parents in children's psychological development, *Pediatrics*, 104, 164, 1999.
71. Maffeis, C., Talamini, G., and Tato, L., Influence of diet, physical activity and parents' obesity on children's adiposity: a four-year longitudinal study, *Int. J. Obes.*, 22, 758, 1998.
72. Darling, N. and Steinbery, L., Parenting style as context: an integrative model, *Psychol. Bull.*, 113, 487, 1993.
73. Pliner, P. and Pelchat, M.L., Similarities in food preferences between children and their siblings and parents, *Appetite*, 7, 333, 1986.
74. Birch, L.L., Zimmerman, S., and Hind, H., The influence of social-affective content on preschool children's food preferences, *Child Dev.*, 51, 856, 1980.
75. Laskarezewski, P. et al., Lipid and lipoprotein tracking in 108 children over a four-year period, *Pediatrics*, 64, 584, 1979.
76. Patterson, T.L. et al., Aggregation of dietary calories, fats and sodium in Mexican-American and Anglo families, *Am. J. Prev. Med.*, 4, 75, 1988.
77. Golan, M., Fairaru, M., and Weizman, A., Role of behavior modification in the treatment of childhood obesity with the parents as the exclusive agents of change, *Int. J. Obes.*, 22, 1217, 1998.
78. Golan, M. et al., Parents as the exclusive agents of change in the treatment of childhood obesity, *Am. J. Clin. Nutr.*, 67, 1130, 1998.
79. Perry, C.L. et al., Changing fruit and vegetable consumption among children the 5-a-Day Power Plus program in St. Paul, Minnesota, *Am. J. Public Health*, 88, 603, 1998.
80. Epstein, L.H. et al., Ten-year follow-up of behavioral, family-based treatment for obese children, *JAMA*, 264, 5219, 1990.
81. St. Jeor, S.T. et al., Family-based interventions for the treatment of childhood obesity, *J. Am. Diet. Assoc.*, 102, 640, 2002.
82. Williams, C.L. et al., Healthy Start: A comprehensive health education program for preschool children, *Prev. Med.*, 27, 216, 1998.
83. Haire-Joshu, D. et al., Improving dietary behavior in African Americans: the Parents as Teachers High 5, Low Fat Program, *Prev. Med.*, 36, 684, 2003.
84. DISC Collaborative Research Group, Efficacy and safety of lowering dietary intake of total fat, saturated fat, and cholesterol in children with elevated LDL-cholesterol: The Dietary Intervention Study in Children (DISC), *JAMA*, 273, 1429, 1995.
85. Berg-Smith, S.M. et al., A brief motivational-intervention to improve dietary adherence in adolescents, *Health Education Research*, 14, 399, 1999.
86. Snetselaar, L. et al., Adolescents eating diets rich in either lean beef or lean poultry and fish reduced fat and saturated fat intake and those eating beef maintained serum ferritin status, *J. Am. Diet. Assoc.*, 104, 424, 2004.
87. The Diabetes Control and Complications Trial Research Group, The effect of intensive treatment of diabetes on the development and progression of long-term complications in insulin-dependent diabetes mellitus, *N. Engl. J. Med.*, 329, 977, 1993.
88. The DCCT Research Group, Nutrition interventions for intensive therapy in the Diabetes Control and Complications Trial, *J. Am. Diet. Assoc.*, 93, 768, 1993.
89. Lipid Research Clinics Program, The Lipid Research Clinics Coronary Primary Prevention Trial Results. I. Reduction in incidence of coronary heart disease, *JAMA*, 251, 351, 1984.

90. Lipid Research Clinics Program, The Lipid Research Clinics Coronary Primary Prevention Trial Results. II. The relationship of reduction in incidence of coronary heart disease to cholesterol lowering, *JAMA*, 251, 365, 1984.
91. Klahr, S. et al., For the Modification of Diet in Renal Disease Study Group, the effects of dietary protein restriction and blood-pressure control on the progression of chronic renal disease, *N. Engl. J. Med.*, 330, 878, 1994.
92. Milas, N.C., Nowalk, M.P., Akpele, L., Costaldo, L., Coyne, T., Doreshenko, L., Kiquwa, L., Korzec-Ramirez, D., Scherch, L.K., and Snetselaar, L., Factors associated with adherence to dietary protein intervention in the Modification of Diet in Renal Disease Study, 95, 1295, 1995.
93. Bowen, D. et al., Results of adjunct dietary intervention program in the Women's Health Initiative, *J. Am. Diet. Assoc.*, 102, 1631, 2002.
94. Howard, B.V., Van Horn, L., Hsia, J., Manson, J.E., Stefanick, M.L., Wasstertheil-Smoller, S., Kuller, L., LaCroix, A.Z., Langer, R.D., Lasser, N.L., Lewis, C.E., Limacher, M.C., Margolis, K.L., Mysiw, W.J., Ockene, J.K., Parker, L.M., Perri, M.G., Phillips, L., Prentice, R.L., Robbins, J., Rossouw, J.E., Sarto, G.E., Schatz, I.J., Snetselaar, L.G. et al., Low-fat dietary pattern and risk of cardiovascular disease: The Women's Health Initiative Randomized Controlled Dietary Modification Trial, *JAMA*, 295, 655–666, 2006.
95. Winters, B.L., Mitchell, D.C., Smiciklas-Wright, H., Grosvenor, M.B., Liu, W., and Blackburn, G.L., Dietary patterns in women treated for breast cancer who successfully reduce fat intake: The Women's Intervention Nutrition Study (WINS), *J. Am. Diet. Assoc.*, 104, 551, 2004.

3

PREDICTORS OF MAINTAINED BEHAVIOR CHANGE WITH EMPHASIS ON WEIGHT LOSS

Michael Perri provides a very eloquent discussion on the topic of ways to maintain adherence specifically in the treatment of obesity [1]. This chapter highlights some of the salient points he makes and applies them to dietary adherence maintenance.

Perri describes several strategies to improve long-term adherence. All of these strategies might potentially be helpful in maintaining long-term adherence to dietary eating patterns and foster lifestyle change. The strategies include a variety of researched approaches: "extended treatment, skills training, monetary incentives, food provision, telephone prompts, peer support, exercise and multi-component maintenance programs" [1].

3.1 EXTENDED TREATMENT

In the effort to reduce the impact of the obesity epidemic, researchers have tried many strategies to optimize weight maintenance. One of the strategies is simply extending the length of time the counselor has in contact with the patient. Perri has researched this concept of extended treatment by comparing a usual care 20-week treatment period with an extended 40-week treatment period [2]. He found that during the period between 20 and 40 weeks, adherence to diet and weight loss continued. Without intervention beyond 40 weeks, weight loss and adherence were not maintained.

Some research studies have included control groups where the initial course of behavioral therapy was 20 weeks, an often-used period of time in many weight loss treatment programs [2–4]. This control period was compared to an extended period of 1 year including the same behavioral therapy. The results of the studies show that the extended treatment group had mean net weight losses of 11.3 kg. Most importantly, the extended care groups were able to maintain 101.6% of the weight they had initially lost in the first 6 months. In comparison, the controls had mean net weight losses of only 6.6 kg and maintained only 66.6% of their initial weight reduction.

Five studies maintained an assessment phase without counselor contact for an average of 21 months [4–8]. Extended treatment showed mean net losses of 8.4 kg and 73.2% of the initial 6-month weight reduction. For the group without extended care, the mean net weight losses were only 3.8 kg and 38.3% of their initial 6-month weight loss. As a group, these studies certainly show the importance of extended behavioral therapy in terms of maintenance of weight reductions. It is important to note that the extended treatment did not result in additional weight loss but rather seemed to help in weight maintenance.

The message we can take from this research is that, in dietary counseling, length of time spent in contact with the patient is crucial. As we plan for treatment programs specifically focused on weight loss, nutrition counselors might carefully design extended contacts that mirror the needs of the patient or groups of patients. For example, for an elderly woman who has just lost her husband, contacts might focus on ways to make the goals she has set easier to follow. This means negotiating with her to assure that any lifestyle changes now work into her existing daily schedule. Cooking for one as opposed to two requires skills and new ways of looking at meal preparation and table setting. Often someone who has lost a spouse will avoid sitting at the table to eat and substitute the behavior of grazing on small amounts of food throughout the day. Changing this one behavior and focusing on it in extended contacts will help bring the patient back to a more healthful eating style.

3.2 SKILLS TRAINING

One of the many skills that is important in lifestyle change is the skill of avoiding the "I quit" scenario. In this scenario the patient sees slight failures or slips as devastating and a signal to end dietary intervention. Several studies have emphasized the concept of relapse prevention training (RPT) as a way of interjecting self-management as a patient struggles with slips in dietary adherence. The goal in RPT is to either avoid or use coping skills to deal with a relapse in lifestyle change behaviors [9].

Baum and his colleagues studied weight loss and found that persons in a minimal contact maintenance condition experienced a significant relapse resulting in weight regain [10]. These researchers then compared this group of more usual care participants to those who were trained in RPT skills in addition to receiving post-treatment contacts and found that they maintained their weight losses. In a similar fashion, Perri and Nezu trained participants in the skill of RPT as part of a multicomponent program of patient–therapist contacts by mail and phone [11]. With this RPT skill addition, weight loss was maintained in follow-up compared to the initial treatment without follow-up sessions.

In work with patients where long-term maintenance is key, nutrition counselors might assure that a session on RPT skills training is provided and that this same thought process of replacing negative with positive thoughts is reinforced during extended contacts. For example, a mother who is trying to provide her young toddler with healthy meals says that she is "just about to give up." Mealtime is always a battleground of her toddler refusing food and her forcing the food upon him. An important concept to keep in mind when dealing with toddlers is that they often are as calm as the parent seems. Parent fears become their fears, and the parent's heightened emotions will be mirrored in their child's reactions. The goal of making mealtime fun for both parent and child is key to successful healthy eating. However, there will be times when a mother cannot control her emotions, and the resulting toddler tantrum is inevitable. The skill of RPT shows the mother that one time where eating around the table reverts to a war zone is not a problem. Mothers can learn from this relapse how important their method of dealing with a problem is to a toddler's behavior. This important lesson is a positive way of coping with relapse. Reminding a mother of the normalcy of not always being in control of her emotions in follow-up phone calls can be very helpful in assuring that the "I give up" scenario need not be an option.

In summary, often patients will take a kind of all-or-nothing approach to lifestyle change. This is a sure setup for failure. It is important that the nutrition counselor identify this behavior early in the counseling process so it can be a focus as extended counseling proceeds.

3.3 FOOD PROVISION

Many studies today use the concept of total or partial feeding to assist patients in following a dietary regimen. The Study of Nutrition in Teens is an example of a partial feeding study where parents and teens were involved in a 3-month program designed to reduce the fat in their diets and determine the level of ferritin in diets that used beef or poultry and fish as a protein source [12]. In this study parents came to a store set up in the school where low-fat foods were offered that fit into each study eating pattern. Parents could choose from a variety of selections that would allow them to feed the entire family for three nights out of a week. Additionally, they attended classes one night a week where a meal was provided for the entire family. This example of food provision allowed participants in the study to self-select some of their meals with the nutritionist controlling a portion of the foods that were eaten in a day.

Jeffery and his colleagues tested the concept of food provision in a weight-loss study [13]. Participants in the study were given prepackaged, portion-controlled, low-calorie meals. Those persons in this study who were given those meals showed greater weight loss than those who were not given meals and needed to totally self-select foods. This difference was maintained throughout the 12-month maintenance phase, but in an additional 1-year follow-up period, weight loss was not maintained [14].

Wing and her associates studied the effectiveness of following a completed behavioral treatment program with an optional offer to purchase prepackaged, portion-controlled, low-calorie meals [15]. Results showed that participants in the study did not purchase the prepackaged foods and this maintenance strategy was not effective.

In studies where the efficacy of a dietary treatment is important, partial or total feeding is important. This type of study often requires limited time to show changes in biological parameters, such as urinary protein [12] and weight loss and blood pressure [16].

In a study designed to look at adherence to diet in terms of self-report compared to total feeding, we found that, when looking at protein intake, it is often difficult for patients to determine what amount of protein a food might contain [12]. For example, determining the cut of meat can make a major difference in the amount of protein eaten (10 g vs. 6 g). By providing all food for an entire study period and analyzing that food for protein content, it is possible to match food eaten with urinary nitrogen excretion. This study showed the difference in self-report for protein and direct analysis of food eaten. In this case, a patient might be told that he or she is not following the diet, when they indeed are but may not have the tools to be as accurate in self-reporting as needed. Nutrition counselors need to take this factor of level of accuracy humanly attainable into account as they evaluate compliance to diet where self-report is one of the only measures of adherence.

Similarly the DASH study was a total feeding study that provided data to indicate how dietary changes result in weight loss and reduced blood pressures levels [16]. The study showed that by giving subjects meals to eat that were rich in fruits, vegetables, and low-fat dairy foods, with reduced saturated and total fat, blood pressure could be substantially lowered. In this crossover study design, 459 adults with systolic blood pressures of less than 160 mm Hg and diastolic blood pressures of 80 to 95 mm Hg were fed a control diet (low in fruits, vegetables, and dairy products, with a fat content typical of the average diet in the U.S.) for 3 weeks. Following this control period participants in the DASH study were randomly assigned for 8 weeks to a control diet, a diet rich in fruits and vegetables, or a "combination" diet rich in fruits, vegetables, and low-saturated fat dairy products and with reduced saturated and total fat. The diet was not reduced in sodium but rather the sodium intake and body weight were held constant during the 8-week study period.

In general, partial and total feeding studies have a place in showing the ability to connect diet and biological markers, but for long-term maintenance of dietary change studies show that they are not successful.

3.4 MONETARY INCENTIVES

Jeffery and his colleagues also studied the effect of monetary incentives on weight-loss maintenance [13]. These researchers looked at the use of money as an incentive along with provision of food and monetary incentives alone. The results showed that just the reward of money made no significant difference in weight loss and weight-loss maintenance.

3.5 TELEPHONE PROMPTS AND COUNSELING

Wing and her associates looked at a very streamlined way of prompting participants to follow their diet [15]. Telephone prompts were designed to merely remind participants to complete self-monitoring forms that tracked lifestyle change behaviors. The persons who called each participant were interviewers who were unknown to the participant. No counseling or advice was given to the participant; the call was merely a reminder. Results of this intervention showed that there was no improvement in weight maintenance with these reminder calls.

University of Iowa nutritionists have begun an intensive process of counseling persons who are very overweight in an industry wellness program. Their work includes the use of motivational interviewing with behavioral and cognitive therapy strategies. While the data relative to change has not been analyzed, initial participant response has been positive, and in roughly a third of the persons participating, weight loss has been achieved. We need additional research in this area of telephone counseling for dietary lifestyle change.

3.6 PEER SUPPORT

We often look at the importance of a buddy or support person as we work with maintenance of diet. A few studies are available to indicate the effects of peer support on adherence and weight loss. Perri and his coworkers devised a study that focused on peer support programs in which participants were taught the skill of running their own support meetings [3]. Each group was given a meeting place equipped with a scale. The intervention involved an initial treatment program with biweekly peer meetings scheduled over a 7-month period. Although attendance rates reached 67%, this peer group support compared to a no-maintenance intervention option resulted in no change in either group in terms of adherence and weight change. In fact, there was a significant weight gain in both groups with the only positive being that the peer support group had a greater mean net weight loss.

There is some controversy over the benefits of recruiting participants who are friends and can be supportive of one another as a lifestyle intervention proceeds. Anecdotally, if two friends join an intervention where dietary change is important, and if one of the duo decides to stop the intervention, often the other partner will do likewise. This scenario has been repeated numerous times in long-term studies where there is a negative result for dietary adherence and retention.

Wing and Jeffery tested this idea in a situation where the hypothesis dealt with recruiting participants with friends to compare them with a standard behavior treatment where persons were recruited alone [17]. The results showed that for those who were recruited with a friend, weight maintenance after 6 months was 66% compared to only 24% of the standard treatment where persons were recruited alone. It is important to carefully assess these results. It seems that the benefits of peer support interventions might be limited to individuals who enter treatment with a partner.

3.7 EXERCISE

Where weight loss is concerned, the equation for weight gain includes both energy intake and output. To maximize success, both need to be a part of intervention where weight loss is the goal. Observational studies using correlational analysis point to the importance of increased exercise or physical activity for long-term weight loss [18]. Additionally, as we look at studies where obese persons have maintained long-term weight loss, exercise is one of the key factors in the maintained behavior change [19]. As we look at controlled trials, it is apparent that few of them show that the combination of exercise plus diet results in significantly greater long-term weight loss compared to diet alone. Perri indicated that the key element here is that often adherence to an exercise regimen is poor [1].

Perri and his coworkers showed that there is a significant difference in home-based vs. group exercise regimens [5]. Following 6 months of exercise intervention, both groups showed significant changes in cardio-respiratory fitness, eating patterns, and weight loss. However, in terms of long-term maintenance of exercise participation and treatment adherence at 1 year of follow-up, the home-based group was superior in number of sessions completed and amount of weight loss achieved and maintained.

It is important in working with both diet and exercise to keep in mind that inclusion of both elements does not mean ultimate weight-loss success. What we can learn from research is that exercise seems to work best when tied to usual life events when modifying lifestyle. Just as diet must be tailored to past eating habits, exercise additions to lifestyle seem to achieve the most positive change relative to maintenance if they are home-based and designed to fit into a usual lifestyle. For adults who are doing well with diet but having problems with weight loss, designing a program of exercise that includes daily walks in a specified area around his home might be one home-based strategy that allows for ease in lifestyle modification.

3.8 MULTICOMPONENT MAINTENANCE PROGRAMS

Research by Perri and his colleagues defined a multicomponent program as one that includes peer group meetings in addition to ongoing contacts by mail and phone [20]. In this skills-building intervention patients were taught to lead their own peer groups and were given postcards on which to self-monitor food intake. The participants in this group were also taught weight-loss strategies to help facilitate weight loss.

This multicomponent intervention was compared to one where participants received initial treatment plus six biweekly booster sessions. The results of the study showed that weight loss both at the end of the maintenance phase and at additional follow-up 6 months later was significantly better in the multicomponent program.

In an attempt to look at exercise as part of the multicomponent program, Perri and his coworkers modified the program above to include a longer initial treatment period of 20 weeks vs. the previous study using 14 weeks [21]. The addition of group-based aerobic exercise resulted in greater weight loss at post-intervention follow-up data collection points.

For one study, Perri and his colleagues designed five interventions [4]:

1. Behavioral therapy alone
2. Behavioral therapy plus extended contact
3. Behavioral therapy plus extended contact plus social influence
4. Behavioral therapy plus extended contact plus aerobic exercise program
5. Behavioral therapy plus extended contact plus aerobic exercise program plus social influence program

The results of this comparison of five interventions were that all four programs compared to the behavioral therapy alone without post-treatment contact showed greater maintenance of weight losses. There were no significant between-group effects for the exercise and social influence groups. However, significant weight loss was observed in the group that received counselor contacts combined with both increased aerobic exercise and the social influence program. A mean net weight loss of 4.1 kg was achieved during the first 6 months of the maintenance phase. The effectiveness of the therapist contact programs was noted with the most significance in the first 6 months of the maintenance phase. Six months after the post-treatment ended, the four maintenance groups succeeded in retaining 70 to 99% of their initial weight losses. In the groups without post-treatment counselor contact only 33% of initial weight loss was maintained.

For the nutrition counselor, use of this research data means extending contact, particularly in the first 6 months of the maintenance phase. Post-treatment contact is a key to successful weight loss. In Perri's program, where multicomponent therapy was used, the sessions occurred biweekly for 26 weeks [4]. A major reason for maintenance of weight loss is patient–counselor contact. This should be the focus of all interventions where lifestyle change is the goal.

There are limitations to extended treatment. Continued counseling is labor intensive and costly. A second issue of concern is the motivation of patients during extended counseling. As treatment duration reaches 1 year, patient attendance to sessions drops off, adherence to diet lapses, and patients often gain weight even though counseling continues. A crucial part of counseling is assuring the patient that expectations might need to be more realistic. Often if goals are too high relative to the amount of weight loss that a program can provide, patients become impatient with a plateau that will result during the extended treatment phase. Adherence will drop as unmet expectations force the patient to rethink the worth of working too hard to reduce pounds with no results. During extended treatment, additional strategies might be needed to increase motivation for extended nutrition counseling. Chapters 7, 8, and 9 provide counseling scripts using motivational interviewing. These methods of increasing adherence have been used in several studies including NIH-funded long-term randomized clinical trials (Diet Intervention Study in Children [22], Study of Nutrition in Teens [23], TREK, Women's Intervention Nutrition Study [24] and Women's Health Initiative [25]). Also, Perri and his colleagues have used strategies focusing on social influence that have increased adherence but not weight loss [4]. Two of those strategies include the following: "learning by teaching," where patients are taught to prepare and deliver weight loss maintenance strategies to their peers, and "telephone networking," which involves planned phone calls focused on providing peer support between in-person sessions.

Perri cautions that extended counseling does not appear to be a strategy that is helpful if large amounts of weight loss are needed where severe energy restriction is a cause of obesity [1]. It is most effective in situations where 6 to 12 kg weight losses are the maintenance goals.

It is always important to focus goals on behaviors within the control of the patients. How much weight they lose is not in their control and will set the patients up for failure. Identifying a type of food and a quantity as a goal is important. For example, one of my patients admitted to eating a candy bar nearly every day. She also knew that the candy bar was the equivalent of about 280 calories. I cautioned her against totally eliminating the candy bar because it might send her into a position of all or nothing where she refused to do a treatment that eliminated a behavior she was incapable of giving up totally. Her goal became one of eating a candy bar only 3 days out of a week. Gradually, the behavior was extinguished completely, but as a counselor I was patient and requested her patience in slowly changing this habit that was difficult to modify.

The one goal we are ultimately striving for might not be the most important goal to change. The Diabetes Prevention Program (DPP) showed that a weight loss of only 7% modified the risk of Type 2 diabetes by 58% in a lifestyle change program [26, 27]. In the REACH study where patients with impaired glucose tolerance were counseled in making lifestyle changes with a focus on eating patterns and exercise, we saw little weight change but significant differences in serum lipids and blood glucose levels [28]. Additional changes may be seen in other areas such as binge eating and depression. All are secondary to the ultimate goal of weight loss but have major effects on overall wellness. It is important to add several measures of success when designing weight-loss programs. For example, reductions in saturated fat can affect coronary heart disease status and assist in weight loss [29]. Likewise, increased physical activity can affect cardio-respiratory health irrespective of weight loss [30].

REFERENCES

1. Perri, M.G., Obese populations, in *Compliance in Healthcare and Research,* Burke, L.E. and Ockene, I.S., eds., Armonk, NY: Futura, 2001, Chap. 13.
2. Perri, M.G. et al., Effect of length of treatment on weight loss, *J. Consult. Clin. Psychol.,* 57, 450, 1989.
3. Perri, M.G. et al., Effects of peer support and therapist contact on long-term weight loss, *J. Consult. Clin. Psychol.,* 55, 615, 1987.
4. Perri, M.G. et al., Effects of four maintenance programs on the long-term management of obesity, *J. Consult. Clin. Psychol.,* 56, 529, 1988.

5. Perri, M.G. et al., Effects of group- versus home-based exercise in the treatment of obesity, *J. Consult. Clin. Psychol.*, 65, 278, 1997.

6. Viegener, B.J. et al., Effects of an intermittent, low-fat, low-calorie diet in the behavioral treatment of obesity, *Behav. Ther.*, 21, 499, 1990.

7. Walden, T.A. et al., Exercise in the treatment of obesity: Effects of four interventions on body composition, resting energy expenditure, appetite, and mood, *J. Consult. Clin. Psychol.*, 65, 269, 1997.

8. Dwing, R.R. et al., Year-long weight loss treatment for obese patients with type II diabetes: does including an intermittent very-low calorie diet improve outcome? *Am. J. Med.*, 97, 354, 1994.

9. Marlatt, G.A. and Gordon, J.R., *Relapse Prevention,* New York: Guilford Press, 1985.

10. Baum, J.G., Clark, H.B., and Sandler, J., Preventing relapse in obesity through post-treatment maintenance systems: comparing the relative efficacy of two levels of therapist support, *J. Behav. Med.*, 14, 287, 1991.

11. Perri, M.G. and Nezu, A.M., Can weight loss be maintained? The effects of post-treatment programs, *Ann. Behav. Med.*, 20, S60, 1998.

12. Snetselaar, L. et al., Protein calculation from food diaries of adult humans underestimates values determined using a biological marker, *J. Nutr.*, 125, 2333, 1995.

13. Jeffery, R.W. et al., Strengthening behavioral interventions for weight loss: a randomized trial of food provision and monetary incentives, *J. Consult. Clin. Psychol.*, 61, 1038, 1993.

14. Jeffery, R.W. and Wing, R.R., Long-term effects of interventions for weight loss using food provision and monetary incentives, *J. Consult. Clin. Psychol.*, 63, 793, 1995.

15. Wing, R.R. et al., Effect of frequent phone contacts and optional food provision on the maintenance of weight loss, *Ann. Behav. Med.*, 18, 172, 1996.

16. Appel, L.J. et al., A clinical trial of the effects of dietary patterns on blood pressure, *N. Engl. J. Med.*, 336, 1117, 1997.

17. Wing, R.R. and Jeffery, R.W., Benefits of recruiting participants with friends and increasing social support for weight loss and maintenance, *J. Consult. Clin. Psychol.*, 67, 132, 1999.

18. Kayman, S., Bruvold, W., and Stern, J.S., Maintenance and relapse after weight loss in women: behavioral aspects, *Am. J. Clin. Nutr.*, 52, 800, 1990.

19. McGuire, M.T. et al., Long-term maintenance of weight loss: do people who lose weight through various weight loss methods use different behaviors to maintain their weight?, *Int. J. Obesity*, 22, 572, 1998.

20. Perri, M.G. et al., Effect of a multi-component maintenance program on long-term weight loss, *J. Consult. Clin. Psychol.*, 52, 480, 1984.

21. Perri, M.G. et al., Enhancing the efficacy of behavior therapy for obesity: effects of aerobic exercise and a multi-component maintenance program, *J. Consult. Clin. Psychol.*, 54, 670, 1986.

22. DISC Collaborative Research Group, Efficacy and safety of lowering dietary intake of total fat, saturated fat, and cholesterol in children with elevated LDL-cholesterol: the Dietary Intervention Study in Children (DISC), *JAMA*, 273, 1429, 1995.

23. Snetselaar, L. et al., Adolescents eating diets rich in either lean beef or lean poultry and fish reduced fat and saturated fat intake and those eating beef maintained serum ferritin status, *J. Am. Diet. Assoc.*, 104, 424, 2004.

24. Winters, B.L., Mitchell, D.C., Smiciklas-Wright, H., Grosvenor, M.B., Liu, W., and Blackburn, G.L., Dietary patterns in women treated for breast cancer who successfully reduce fat intake: The Women's Intervention Nutrition Study (WINS), *J. Am. Diet. Assoc.*, 104, 551, 2004.

25. Bowen, D. et al., Results of adjunct dietary intervention program in the Women's Health Initiative, *J. Am. Diet. Assoc.*, 102, 1631, 2002.

26. The Diabetes Prevention Program (DPP) Research Group, The Diabetes Prevention Program (DPP): description of lifestyle intervention, *Diabetes Care,* 25, 2165, 2002.

27. Nathan, D.M. and Delahanty, L.M., *Beating Diabetes,* New York: McGraw-Hill, 2005.

28. Snetselaar, L.G., unpublished data, 2006.

29. Insull, W. et al., Results of a feasibility study of a low-fat diet, *Arch. Int. Med.,* 150, 421, 1990.

30. Paffenbarger, R.S. and Lee, I.M., Physical activity and fitness for health and longevity, *Res. Q. Exerc. Sport,* 67, 11, 1996.

4

LIFESTYLE CHANGE FACTORS RELATED TO LIFECYCLE STAGES 1, 2, AND 3

4.1 STAGE 1: CHILDHOOD AND PARENTAL FEEDING HABITS

For children the key to prevention of poor eating habits resides in the hands of the parents who are procuring, preparing, and serving the food. The strategies below are designed to include educational, motivational, behavioral, and cognitive change theories. To help in assuring appropriate strategies, it is important for parents to embrace learning new strategies and changing existing unhealthy behaviors so that they are not passed down to future generations.

For children less than 2 years of age, the emphasis is on introducing solid foods at the appropriate developmental stage and later expanding food variety (see Appendix A). The USDA Food Guide Pyramid for Young Children provides dietary guidelines for children 2 and older, with a focus on fruits and vegetables (www.healthierus.gov/dietaryguidelines).

Baranowski and his colleagues reviewed psychological factors related to dietary intake for interventions involving nutrition-related lifestyle change [1]. They point out that no single theory provided models that regularly out-predicted others in terms of dietary behaviors such as fruit and vegetable consumption, and they emphasize the importance of combining theories in dietary interventions. Using education and behavior change strategies involves multiple theories and concepts that drive dietary intervention. Figure 4.1 provides an illustrated view of the differences in education and behavior change.

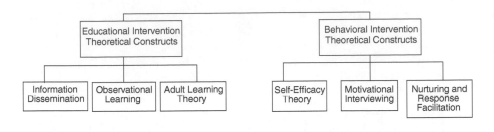

Figure 4.1 Theories and concepts including education and behavioral change.

4.1.1 Educational Dietary Intervention Aspects

4.1.1.1 Overview

The educational aspects of the dietary intervention are designed to present nutrition information to parents in a traditional style. For example, the focus might be on increasing fruits and vegetables within the context of the USDA Dietary Guidelines. The educational intervention begins with guidelines appropriate to the pediatric development stage relative to feeding practices and transitions to the USDA Food Guide Pyramid for Young Children at 2 years of age (see Chapter 1).

4.1.1.2 Core Elements

Education might include: (1) the health benefits associated with eating more fruits and vegetables, (2) when and how to introduce fruits and vegetables, (3) creative ways to increase variety and intake, and (4) the importance of parental modeling based on observational learning. These core elements might include the following: group sessions with interactive lectures, food demonstrations, educational handouts, phone calls, e-mails, newsletters, personalized storybooks, games, etc.

4.1.1.3 Theoretical Model

The educational aspect of a dietary intervention may be based on several theoretical concepts, including information dissemination, observational learning, and adult learning principles. These theories are learning-oriented not behavioral change models.

1. Dissemination — Dissemination of information is critical in increasing parental knowledge about childhood nutrition. Parents need information regarding when to introduce solid foods, what foods to introduce, and what foods to avoid to prevent choking hazards [2, 3].

2. Observational learning — Observational learning encourages parents to model appropriate food choices for their child. For example, by eating a wide variety of fruits and vegetables, parents can promote fruits and vegetable consumption in their children [4].
3. Adult learning principles — Knowles' theories form the basis of much of the current adult learning principles. He identifies the following characteristics of adult learners. They are autonomous and self-directed. They have accumulated a foundation of life experiences and knowledge that could be integrated into a dietary intervention through open-ended questioning posed by the nutrition counselor. Adults are goal- and relevancy-oriented. They are practical and need to be shown respect by the counselor through constant checks on their thoughts and ideas. It is important to tailor the dietary intervention to these adult learner characteristics [5] (www.cc.hawaii.edu/intranet/committees/FacDevCom/guidebk/teachtip/adults-2.htm).

4.1.2   Behavioral Change Aspects

4.1.2.1   Overview

The behavioral change aspects of dietary interventions use strategies to assist parents in adopting a feeding style that will promote healthy eating behaviors and self-regulation of food intake in children. This type of dietary intervention offers guidance in not only how to eat more healthy foods, but also focuses on the process of feeding infants as they begin to eat solid foods. The goal in the behavior change for nutrition lifestyle intervention is to facilitate problem solving around the concept of infant feeding practices. The aim would be to alter feeding practices in parents by using behavioral change strategies based on self-efficacy, motivational interviewing, and nurturing concepts, and potentially refocus toward positive coping strategies to deal with parental feelings that are often not addressed in routine counseling sessions.

4.1.2.2   Core Elements

The core elements of an intervention of this type are knowing:

1. how children learn food preferences (exposure, response facilitation, context, and consequences of eating)
2. what normal and adaptive behaviors occur when infants begin eating solid foods
3. why children reject novel foods and prefer others

4. how parental feeding strategies affect their children's ability to self-regulate food intake.

It is important to incorporate these core elements with the following: interactive group sessions using motivational interviewing techniques, role playing, problem solving, and use of a feeding process designed to maximize a child's ability to self-regulate food intake. See http://www.cdc.gov/nccdphp/dnpa/qualitative_research/index.htm for an example of a feeding process-oriented DVD developed by the Centers for Disease Control (CDC). The nutrition counselor might use these concepts when leading discussions on how parents might change their feeding practices.

4.1.2.3 Theoretical Model

The behavioral change aspects of nutrition lifestyle change might be influenced by the following behavioral theories:

1. Self-efficacy theory — Focuses on the parent's ability to succeed [7]. The nutrition counselor assists the parent in feeling confident about making change. The resulting parental optimism in making parental feeding changes has the potential for a high level of success.
2. Motivational interviewing (MI) — Based on the work of Miller and Rollnick, MI emphasizes a client-centered counseling approach to enhance commitment and confidence for behavior change and to help parents explore and resolve ambivalence [8, 9]. This theory has both positive and unequivocal results in children (see Chapter 6). Major principles used in MI include reflective listening that is intended to build empathy for the parent, show discrepancy between the parent's goals and current problems with child feeding practice behavior, and provide objective feedback. Sessions using MI are designed to avoid argumentation by assuming that the parent is responsible for the decision to change and roll with resistance. This technique emphasizes supporting self-efficacy and optimism for change. The MI framework recognizes the concept that readiness to change fluctuates as a product of interpersonal interaction. The intervention relationship functions at its best when the nutrition counselor and parent work as partners rather than as an expert and recipient. Motivation for child feeding behavior change is not imposed by the nutrition counselor but rather elicited from the parent. In this method, parents reflect on past performance and use it to resolve their own ambivalence. The MI process stresses the concept of change through reflective listening skills rather than a drive to give information. The level of detail in the

knowledge we impart is far less important than the level of skill we use in reflective listening.

3. Nurturing concepts including response facilitation — The concept of nurturing evolves from research based on parenting with healthy feeding styles [10–13]. The emphasis is on healthy feeding practices (i.e., refraining from restricting a child's access to food or pressuring a child to eat more food). Therefore, rather than coaxing and bribing children to eat fruits and vegetables, parents will allow their children to be led by their own internal cues to eat, beginning when they first try solid foods. Response facilitation involves more than just observational learning. It includes allowing the child to participate in nutrition-related activities that involve selecting, preparing, and eating a food.

4. Positive coping strategies to deal with parental feelings — Being a parent is a difficult role fraught with a mixture of emotions that fall on opposite ends of the continuum, from joyfulness and love to deepest fear and anger. When this mix of emotions occurs around a child's eating behaviors, parents must stop to accurately identify or tag their emotions and deal with each appropriately. Anger and frustration often surface when children refuse to eat. Coping with this situation might involve thoughts of ways to remain calm and not give in to poor eating behaviors. Trying to balance this negative feeling with one of joy in just having a vibrant healthy child sitting at the dinner table can often turn negative behavior in a child to positive behavior.

4.1.3 Strategies Used to Change Parent/Child Feeding Practices — Contrasting Educational and Behavioral Change Aspects

Table 4.1 illustrates the differences in the educational and behavioral change dietary intervention strategies.

4.1.4 Intervention Development

Scripts for the intervention group sessions may serve as guides to tailor each intervention.

4.2 STAGE 2: REMEDIATION IN CHILDHOOD AND ADOLESCENCE

Many of the same concepts described above apply to Stage 2. Below is a review of methods used in a randomized clinical trial where children and teens were involved. In the Diet Intervention Study in Children (DISC)

Table 4.1 Strategies Used to Change Parental Child Feeding Practices — Contrasting Educational and Behavioral Change Strategies[a]

	Educational Strategies	Behavioral Change Strategies
Group sessions	The intervention nutritionist demonstrates dishes including fruits and vegetables	The intervention nutritionist discusses the parents' past experience with picking, preparing, and eating fruits and vegetables, including their parents' child feeding practice; this takes place as a fruit and vegetable dish is being demonstrated
Telephone call	The intervention nutritionist describes the reasons that fruits and vegetables are nutrient dense and discusses ways to increase their consumption	The intervention nutritionist discusses meal times and uses motivational interviewing techniques to elicit problem child feeding practices and define potential solutions; the nutrition interventionist will discuss feelings related to mealtimes and ways to deal with those feelings
Tailored storybooks	The storybook includes the child's name within fun stories that include parents encouraging children to eat fruits and vegetables, assigning a very positive quality to the nutrients in them	The storybook includes the child's name within fun stories that illustrate children making their own decisions about picking, preparing, and eating fruits and vegetables
One-page newsletter	The newsletter includes the child's name and has fun recipes that include fruits and vegetables	The newsletter includes the child's name and illustrates how parents and children can work together in picking, preparing, and eating fruits and vegetables

[a] Specific sessions for education and behavior change appear in Appendix B and C.

we used a brief motivational intervention model to enhance dietary adherence with adolescents [14]. In the first three years of this study, children participated in a family-based group intervention designed to modify dietary choices with an emphasis on reducing saturated fat in foods eaten. As these children moved into adolescence, adherence to dietary changes became much more difficult. Peers became dictators of dietary choices, and pressure to eat less healthy foods was the norm. Also, as teens made decisions, parental influence became a more negative and less positive force. To address dietary adherence as children entered teenage years, nutrition counselors implemented an individual-level motivational intervention. This intervention model was based on several theoretical constructs including stages of change [15, 16], motivational interviewing [17], brief negotiation [18], and behavioral self-management [19]. During DISC, a preliminary test of this multifaceted method in teens provided positive results in several areas. It was an appropriate addition to the original family-based group intervention and proved to be acceptable to teens and well-received by nutrition counselors.

This methodology, which includes brief motivational interventions, seems particularly appropriate for the adolescent stage of life with a focus on prevention relative to health factors. Several reasons exist for the compatibility of this model with the adolescent developmental stage. First, dangers surrounding most adolescents are related to social and behavioral factors, including substance abuse, accidents, sexually transmitted diseases, eating disorders, and depression [20–23]. A key to providing the message that an adolescent is not invincible lies with health care professionals. They are the primary conveyors of lifesaving information in a "teachable moment" for teens. A 1994 report of the Surgeon General indicates that adolescents view health professionals above parents and other adults as credible.

Second, as we look at this developmental stage, adolescents are in an exploratory phase where they often initiate participation in health-compromising behaviors [25]. Werch and his colleagues describe the connection between stages of behavior initiation and stages of change model [26]. Other researchers describe the benefit of motivational interviewing during early stages of health behavior change [27, 28].

Third, a primary aim during adolescence is the desire to establish an independent identity separate from family, parents, and other adults. Peers become the group targeted for approval rather than authoritarian adults [29]. The motivational interviewing style provides teens with an increased sense of lifestyle control [30]. The brief intervention model inherent in motivational interviewing includes elements of tailoring to a teen's unique goals, circumstances, and readiness to change [30].

Berg-Smith describes the course of a potential intervention in the last chapter, Figure 14.1. (This schematic has been used in many age groups and appears at the end of the text as a summary.) This process worked well during dietary intervention sessions with teens in the DISC program [14]. Using this process allowed for varying stages of readiness to change and feasible time-limited encounters (5 to 30 min). Also it was adaptable for in-person and telephone dietary intervention sessions.

Adolescence is a time when emotions can run high. When nutrition lifestyle change is needed, feelings are often a major reason for lack of dietary adherence. Teaching an adolescent how to tag feelings might be a beginning to changing unhealthy dietary behaviors. Learning how to appropriately respond to feelings, such as crying when sad instead of eating, may be an important skill learned in adolescence and carried into adulthood.

4.3 STAGE 3: REMEDIATION IN ADULTS AND THE ELDERLY

A similar study in the Women's Health Initiative (WHI) was done using motivational interviewing techniques in elderly women [31]. In this ancillary study WHI participants were involved in three steps of motivational interviewing: assessment, intervention, and future directions. The assessment step focused on identifying the participant's current desire to make further changes. Each participant was assigned to one of three intervention phases: Phase 1 — not ready to change; Phase 2 —unsure about change; Phase 3 — ready to change.

In Phase 1 (not ready to change) the goals for the participant included the following:

1. Increasing awareness of the importance of changing dietary behaviors
2. Identifying and reducing the barriers to healthy eating habits
3. Increasing interest in considering steps toward dietary change

The participant was asked to describe what would need to be different to move forward and to identify sources of barriers to dietary change.

In Phase 2 (unsure about change) the goal was to build readiness to change. In this phase the participant was asked to list the positive and negative aspects of changing eating habits, imagine how life could be different after change, and estimate problems and successes after those changes were made. A key element for the nutrition counselor was to avoid assuming the participant was ready to change. This assumption could lead to feelings of failure.

During Phase 3 (ready to change) the goal was to work with the participant to design an action plan for dietary change that would allow success. The WHI participant was asked to set feasible short-term goals while developing the action plan. Chapter 7 provides additional information on this WHI ancillary study and use of MI in achieving dietary change.

In adults and the elderly, tagging feelings might be an important step to assuring nutrition lifestyle change. In busy adults dietary changes might seem impossible due to overwhelming schedules that are often not in their control. This can lead to frustration and an all-or-nothing attitude that allows maladaptive coping skills (i.e., eating in an unhealthy manner). By appropriately tagging a feeling as guilt, it is possible to refocus priorities on eating as a family to allow for more healthy foods.

The elderly, who often have the stresses of aging when friends' and relatives' illnesses become a priority, might benefit from the strategy of focusing on feelings and responses to those feelings. To identify stress with the specific feeling of sadness and cope with the appropriate emotional release of crying might help with stopping the maladaptive coping mechanism of eating in an unhealthy way.

Each of the lifecycle stages poses new problems with achievement of dietary change. Given these differences there are still many similarities in the path a nutrition counselor takes to facilitate success. Chapters 5, 6, and 7 focus on each stage and provide examples of counseling strategies.

REFERENCES

1. Baranowski, T., Cullen, K.W., and Baranowski, J., Psychosocial correlates of dietary intake: advancing intervention, *Annu. Rev. Public Health*, 19, 17, 1999.
2. Crockett, S.J. et al., Parent education in youth-directed nutrition interventions, *Prev. Med.*, 17, 475, 1989.
3. Pirouznia, M., The association between nutrition knowledge and eating behavior in male and female adolescents in the U.S., *Int. J. Food Sci. Nutr.*, 52, 127, 2001.
4. Harper, L.V. and Sanders, K.M., The effect of adults' eating on young children's acceptance of unfamiliar foods, *J. Exp. Child Psychol.*, 20, 206, 1975.
5. Knowles, M.S., *The Modern Practice of Adult Education: Andragogy vs. Pedagogy*, New York: New York Association Press, 1970.
6. www.cc.hawaii.edu/intranet/committees/FacDevCom/guidebk/teachtip/adults-2.html.
7. Bandura, A., *Self-efficacy: The Exercise of Control*, New York: WH Freeman, 1997.
8. Miller, W.R. and Rollnick, S., *Motivational Interviewing: Preparing People for Change*, New York: Guilford Press, 2002.
9. Prochaska, J.O. et al., Stages of change and decisional balance for twelve problem behaviors, *Health Psychol.*, 13, 39, 1994.
10. Baumrind, D., The influence of parenting style on adolescent competence and substance use, *J. Early Adol.*, 11, 56, 1991.
11. Darling, N. and Steinbery, L., Parenting style as context: an integrative model, *Psychol. Bull.*, 113, 487, 1993.

12. Johnson, S.L. and Birch, L.L., Parents' and children's adiposity and eating style, *Pediatrics*, 94, 653, 1994.
13. Costanzo, P.R. and Woody, E.Z., Domain-specific parenting styles and their impact on the child's development of particular deviance: the example of obesity proneness, *J. Soc. Clin. Psychol.*, 3, 425, 1985.
14. Berg-Smith, S.M. et al., A brief motivational intervention to improve dietary adherence in adolescents, *Health Educ. Res.*, 14, 399–410, 1999.
15. Prochaska, J. and DiClemente, C., Transtheoretical therapy: toward a more integrative model of change, *Psychotherapy: Theory, Research and Practice*, 19, 276, 1982.
16. Prochaska, J. and DiClemente, C., Toward a comprehensive model of change, in *Treating Addictive Behaviors: Processes of Change*, Miller, W.R. and Heather, N., Eds., New York: Plenum, 1986, 3.
17. Miller, W. and Rollnick, S., *Motivational Interviewing: Preparing People to Change Addictive Behaviors*, New York: Guilford Press, 1991.
18. Rollnick, S., Heather, N., and Bell, A., Negotiating behavior change in medical settings: the development of brief motivational interviewing, *J. Mental Health*, 1, 25, 1992.
19. Watson, D.L. and Tharp, R.G., *Self-Directed Behavior: Self-Modification for Personal Adjustment*, 5th ed., Pacific Grove, CA: Brooks/Cole, 1989.
20. Jessor, R., Adolescent development and health behavior, in *Behavioral Health: A Handbook of Health Enhancement and Disease Prevention*, Matarazzo, J., Weiss, S., Herd, J., Miller, N., and Wiss, M., Eds., New York: John Wiley, 1984, 69–90.
21. Erwin, C. and Millstein, S., Biopsycholosocial correlates of risk-taking behaviors in adolescence: can the physician intervene? *J. Adolescence Health Care*, 7 (Suppl.), 82s, 1986.
22. Blum, R., Contemporary threats to adolescent health in the United States, *JAMA*, 257, 3390,1987.
23. Hofmann, A., Clinical assessment and management of health risk behavior in adolescents, *Adolescent Medicine: State of the Art Reviews*, 1, 330, 1989.
24. U.S. Surgeon General, *Preventing Tobacco Use Among Young People*, S/N 7-001-0044 1-0 (DHHS). Washington, DC: U.S. Government Printing Office, 1994.
25. Jaffe, A., Radius, S., and Gall, M., Health counseling for adolescents: what they want, what they get and who gives it, *Pediatrics*, 82, 481,1988.
26. Werch, C.H. and DiClemente, D.D., A multi-component stage model for matching drug prevention strategies and messages to youth stage of use, *Health Educ. Res.*, 9, 37, 1994.
27. Rollnick, S. and Morgan, M., Motivational interviewing: increasing readiness to change, in *Psychotherapy and Substance Abuse: A Practitioner's Handbook*, Washton, A.M., Ed., New York: Guilford Press, 1994, 179–191.
28. Grimley, D. et al., Contraceptive and condom use adoption and maintenance: a stage paradigm approach, *Health Educ. Q.*, 22, 20, 1995.
29. Christopher, J., Nagle, D., and Hansen, D., Social skills interventions with adolescents, *Behav. Modif.*, 17, 314, 1993.
30. Tober, G., Motivational interviewing with young people, in *Motivational Interviewing*, Miller, W.R. and Rollnick, S., Eds., New York: Guilford Press, 1991, 248–259.
31. Bowen, D. et al., Results of an adjunct dietary intervention program in the Women's Health Initiative, *J. Am. Diet. Assoc.*, 102, 1631, 2002.

5

MOTIVATIONAL INTERVIEWING FOR CHILDHOOD AND PARENTAL FEEDING HABITS: STAGE 1

5.1 PARENTAL INFANT FEEDING PRACTICES ASSOCIATED WITH FOOD PREFERENCES

Recent research shows that an infant's food acceptance is associated with flavors in mother's milk or formula. Infants who experienced the flavor of carrots in mother's milk finish eating carrot-flavored cereal more quickly than control infants whose mothers were not eating carrots during lactation [1]. After exposure to carrots or a variety of vegetables, infants ate more of the carrots. Additionally, daily experience with fruit initially increased the infant's willingness to eat carrots [2]. A final study showed that the mothers' reported willingness to eat novel foods and their associated flavors was reflected in their infant's preferences for flavored cereal [3].

Birch and other researchers set out to identify the ways in which children form food preferences [4] and observed that those preferences are associated with parental learning experiences related to food. The determination of preference in young children might be tied to time allowed for experiencing a food. When exposure to a food is repetitive and positive, a continued preference for that food occurs [5–9]. Changes in parental behavior in food selection and preparation are essential to the development of child food preferences that focus on healthful selections.

Often well-meaning parents, in an effort to increase healthy eating, might force food selection in small children. This practice can result in a child's negative preference for those foods [5, 6, 10, 11]. Based on health professionals' recommendations, parents will encourage children to eat more fruits and vegetables. Parents' feedback to children aimed at increasing consumption of vegetables has resulted in a lower preference for vegetables later in life [12].

Observational research shows that parents withhold foods they feel are unhealthy with the intention of forming good eating habits [13, 14]. Research data indicate the negative aspects of using food as a reward, showing subsequent increases in the child's preference for that food [15]. Based on research findings when a parent restricted a food, a child was more likely to eat that food in an "unrestricted" setting, such as a friend's home [5, 6].

Parents are faced with the challenge of altering their children's intake to make food selections more healthful. Food preferences are especially important in determining what is eaten because children eat foods they like and avoid those they dislike [16–20]. Fisher and Birch (1995) showed the importance of food preferences by serving a diet consisting of ~33% of calories from fat to a group of children. After analyzing foods actually eaten by the children, they found that the percent of calories from fat was widely divergent, ranging from 25 to 42% of calories from fat.

Research in toddlers indicates that repeated opportunities to consume new foods will increase preference for and intake of that food [5, 6, 8, 9, 21]. In those studies 5 to 10 exposures were necessary before toddlers responded positively to a food. These findings focus on the importance of early experience with foods to increase acceptance.

Use of internal cues signaled by appetite to eat or stop eating should be encouraged as a focus of parental child feeding practices. Researchers document the direct relationship of appetite-driven intake with total calories eaten [22, 23]. Rewarding children for eating decreases their responsiveness to the energy content of the foods dictated by appetite [7].

In a wonderful book devoted to realistic goals that parents might use in setting the stage for healthful eating practices, Satter discusses an alternate way to control child feeding practices using a division of responsibility. She recommends that the parent be responsible for healthful selection of foods, with an upbeat family-focused eating atmosphere, while the child decides when and how much to eat [24, 25].

5.2 EVALUATING A CHILD'S EATING HABITS

Determining a child's existing eating habits and preferences can be a guide to where change in eating behavior might occur. A variety of methods can be used to evaluate children's eating habits. Van Horn and colleagues describe the DISC experiences where saturated fat intake was targeted and analyzed in children [26]. DISC was one of the first studies to report that children younger than 10 years had the ability to report foods eaten and, with the use of portion pictures, estimated amounts of foods they had eaten [27–32]. Researchers now apply the same techniques used to collect dietary data in adults to children, including a parent's version of their child's intake [33, 34]. One study in school-age children combined parent's observations and the child's recall with resulting complete and accurate dietary intake data [33]. Training to standardize information provided by parent and child results in comparable data gathered from parents' recall and their child's self-report [35].

Counseling parents can be difficult due to intense positive emotions relative to their children and yet an extreme desire to assure that all is perfect relative to eating habits. As a nutrition counselor it is important to understand these mixed emotions and focus on assessing them.

Initially, the assessment involves determining the readiness-to-change level (ready, unsure, not ready). Using a ruler or a scale concept ask, "On a scale of 1 to 12, how ready are you to make dinnertime less of a battle ground? (1 = not ready to change mealtimes; 12 = very ready to change mealtimes)." Most parents will jump to indicate that they are very ready to end the battleground scenario during meals. However many have fallen into the trap of being willing to do anything relative to letting their children eat what they want so that mealtimes are calm and quiet. It is important to recognize that an initial response of 12 might not be as easy as the parent might think. Additionally, assessing whether both parents are ready to change is important. If one parent is willing to try new strategies and the other will do anything to keep mealtimes peaceful even if that means letting the child eat whatever he or she wants, problems in changing the mealtime behavior may occur.

A crucial point to remember is that every counseling session does not have to end with parental agreement to make changes. A decision to think about change is a successful conclusion to a motivational interviewing session.

5.3 NOT-READY-TO-CHANGE COUNSELING SESSION

The not-ready-to-change intervention involves the following three goals:

1. Facilitate the parents' ability to consider change
2. Reduce their resistance to the change after an initial attempt is unsuccessful
3. Identify steps to change mealtimes that are tailored to the family's needs

Family size and eating habits of other children in the family will play a role in the level of change and how quickly that change can occur. The family's level of communication when the dietary intervention begins will play a role in how quickly success can be achieved. Parental expectation for success will determine how quickly they give in to a child's wishes. The parental level of patience with child behavior will also affect the level of success and the rapidity with which positive change in mealtime behavior occurs.

There are several communication skills that will help in achieving the three goals listed above.

Open-ended questions: An open-ended question requires more than a "yes" or "no" answer. It is answered by explaining or discussing. For example:

- "Tell me about how your mealtimes are going."
- "What are the positive aspects of the mealtime changes you have made so far? What problems are connected with making those changes?"

Reflective listening: The nutrition counselor listens in a reflective way as parents identify feelings that surface as they describe particularly difficult mealtimes where behavior-change strategies have been tested. This type of listening is more than just paraphrasing words a parent voices. Reflective listening includes the nutrition counselor's thoughts on what the parent feels and is restated as a statement rather than a question. A parent's true feelings about changes in mealtime battles over a child's eating habits can be determined by using reflection. For example:

Parent: "I am not a very patient person. When Johnny refuses to eat, I feel worried that he will suffer from malnutrition. He doesn't eat enough to keep a fly alive. When I get worried, I tend to be impatient. This is the point at which dinnertime becomes a battle-ground of pushing and shoving relative to eating."

Caregiver: "You feel frustrated because you really want to change what happens at the dinner table but at the same time it requires so much patience to deal with Johnny's eating habits that you give up trying."

Affirming: Parents never want to be labeled as "bad" or "incompetent." The nutrition counselor can play a role in assuring that these labels do not cause the parent to feel defeated. When the nutrition counselor is affirming, he or she is sending the message that parental struggles are normal and occur in all families. With this message of normalcy comes the promise that the nutrition counselor is available in difficult situations when dealing with child eating behaviors seems almost impossible. For example:

- "I know that it is difficult for you to talk with me about this problem you are having with your child at mealtimes, but thank you for making the effort. All of my clients have experienced the problems that you are having."
- "You have had an incredible schedule with three children and a full-time job. I feel that you have done extremely well given your circumstances."
- "A mother I saw yesterday described the same problems. I can understand why you are having difficulty."

Summarizing: Summarizing key concepts discussed around child eating behaviors during the nutrition counseling session assures that the counselor understands issues that are often complex. A simple, concise statement of what you, the nutrition counselor, thought you heard is often helpful.

Eliciting self-motivational statements: The four communication skills described above are important to this final strategy, eliciting self-motivational statements. The goals of these statements to facilitate the parent's realization of what is happening when a child is throwing a temper tantrum during a mealtime are threefold:

1. That a problem exists; for example:
   - "I know that your child is quite familiar with exhibiting a tantrum and being given what he wants, often a dessert. What about this scenario is most problematic for you?"
   - "Tell me, from your point of view as a parent, in what ways has changing the way you deal with your child's eating habits been a problem?"
2. That concern exists about it; for example:
   - "When you give in to your child and feed him only those foods he likes that are high in fat and simple sugar, how do you feel?"
   - "Describe your concerns when you just can't get Johnny to eat those things you feel are healthy for him."
   - "What are your concerns if he never changes the types of foods he is eating?"
3. That in the future, positive steps can be taken to correct the problem; for example:
   - "If you could be assured that Johnny ate in a healthy way all of the time, what would need to be different for you?"
   - "What do you see as advantages to changing Johnny's eating habits?"

- "If you decided to make a change in your mealtimes with Johnny, what would need to happen?"
- "You have done many things in your work that require devotion and dedication. What makes you think that if you decided to make a change with mealtimes and your child's eating behavior that you could do it?"
- "What encourages you that you can change mealtimes if you want to?"
- "If you decided to change, what strategies would help you maintain that change?"

It is important to be tentative when approaching a parent about problem eating behaviors: "Would you be willing to continue our discussion and talk about the possibility of change?"

In order to allow time for a thoughtful discussion around eating habits, ask open-ended questions or command statements.

- "Tell me why you picked _____ on the ruler."
- "What would need to happen for you to move from a 3 to a 12 on the ruler? What might I do to help you get there?"

For a new parent or a seasoned parent attentive nutrition counseling can set the stage for change. Parents need to know that they have done many things well in dealing with their child's eating behaviors. Using summary statements to remind parents of these successes is vital to eventual change. The parent who feels upbeat and in control will be a more positive influence on child eating behaviors. Summary statements that focus on small changes that have happened at the dinner table, such as the child eating a small amount of vegetables as compared to none, are crucial in achieving change. Restating reasons for change can also be very important. Asking a question about what would help the parent move forward might also be advantageous to change. Summarization will allow parents to rethink the rationale for change.

Counselors often strive for goal-setting behaviors in parents who still might not realize the difficulties associated with changing mealtime behaviors. In this stage of change, forcing goal-setting behaviors will only cause feelings of defeat for both the parent and counselor.

"I can understand why this is a difficult time for you to make changes in your eating habits. Just being able to state the problems you are having is a very positive step forward. Things do change in our lives. When you are ready to discuss changes, I am always available. Based on decisions you have made in the past, I know you will come back to me when the time is right."

A crucial topic to cover prior to ending the session is the confidence and hope you have in the parent's ability to make changes. Finally, arrange for a follow-up contact.

5.4 UNSURE-ABOUT-CHANGE COUNSELING SESSIONS

Parents are often unsure about the degree of effort it will take to change their child's eating behavior. In this stage the goal is to build readiness to change, so that major steps can be taken by parents to alter their child's eating behavior. Often the parent is eager to change the way he or she deals with child eating behaviors at the dinner table, but the eagerness changes as the task becomes one where great patience is needed. This stage may occur after a trial at modifying a child's eating behavior. Ambivalence begins to replace eagerness in this stage. For the counselor, this is the time to explore the positive reasons for making the change in the first place. It is also a time to realistically discuss the negatives that have surfaced following strategy testing. For example:

■ "Tell me some of the things you like about the old ways you used to deal with your child's eating behaviors at mealtime."
■ "What were some of the good things you stated earlier that would occur if your child's eating habits changed?"

The nutrition counselor's goal is to help the parent feel confident enough to consider the extra time and effort it will take to change child eating behaviors. In some instances visualizing a scenario where mealtime is fun for the reasons originally determined to be positive about the change can end in desired results. The nutrition counselor might begin with the following statement: "It is very apparent to me that mealtimes have been more difficult in this first try at changing your child's eating behavior. I can understand how this makes you want to give up. Try to think what mealtimes might be like if you were able to make one small change in your child's eating habits. What would your mealtime be like and what specifically would you want to do?" Finally, the nutrition counselor summarizes the positive and negative aspects of strategies used to make mealtime more fun and includes potential plans for change.

Work with parents to set broad goals with specific goals to follow. For example, "How would you like things to be different?" and "What do you want to change?"

Discuss strategies for mealtime changes that would seem to work best for the family. If one is ineffective, another might be perfect for the child's eating behavior change. Parents might write a plan that would include what they intend to do prior to the next nutrition counseling session.

Finally, statements that affirm and encourage are needed. "I will not force you into trying these strategies. You have said that you are unsure. Take your time and know that I am always available to help you."

5.5 READY-TO-CHANGE COUNSELING SESSIONS

In this stage, goal setting is key. The nutrition counselor provides the parent with tools to use in meeting goals.

Helping the parent confirm that change at this time is appropriate is important. Using the ruler again ask, "Why did you choose a 3 instead of a 1 or a 12? Give me some ideas for why you think you are ready to change."

First steps in trying to achieve child eating behavior change are very important. Sometimes parents might feel that it is easier to just continue with poor habits reinforcing a child's eating behavior rather than trying new strategies to modify their child's behavior. The following questions can help in solidifying the idea that a parent is ready to embark on changing what happens at the dinner table. "What specifically could you do to make a change in your child's eating habits? Is this a truly workable plan? How will things be different for you if you make these changes?"

Helping parents work gradually toward changes at mealtimes is vital to eventual success. The nutrition counselor might say, "Let's do things gradually. What is a short-term goal that you know is positioned for success?"

Delineate the specifics that will make it obvious that the goal has been reached. Identify obstacles to success but at the same time carefully identify how to be successful. Early identification of barriers to success will allow for strategies to avoid them and increase the likelihood of success. Work with both parents, if possible, and include roles for other family members in being supportive of changes that will affect the child's eating behavior.

List markers that can be identified during the meal that indicate when strategies are successful. Small successes might not be identified early enough, resulting in the feeling that the plan is just not working. Writing down the plan will help the parent solidify the feasibility of actually carrying out the behavior change strategies.

In closing the nutrition counseling session, offer encouraging statements: "You have made great strides in changing what happens at your family table. At this point you are the expert at what will and will not work for your family. Making a change that involves several members of the family is very difficult. If one strategy does not work, try another. The idea of continuing to try to make changes is important. Eventually you will be successful."

Parents with small children who are having difficulties with eating solid food are very open to accepting advice. This is a period in life that might be referred to as a "teachable moment." However, while some advice is helpful, too much information might result in a lack of action and decision making by parents. Asking at several points in a nutrition counseling session, "What will work best for you?" can be a beneficial way of encouraging parental action without dictation by the nutrition counselor. When the parent feels secure in decision making, strides can be made away from the counseling session to the home setting, where planning and strategizing can make the biggest impact.

5.6 SUMMARY

- Dealing with parents who must make changes in children's eating habits requires an understanding of how the parent deals with other aspects of child behavior.
- Patience is required so that change can occur gradually.
- Encouraging parents who are in a "teachable moment" to make changes with the hope of success can ensure that feelings of defeat are not a final result.

REFERENCES

1. Mennella, J.A. and Beauchamp, G.K., Experience with a flavor in mother's milk modifies the infant acceptance of flavored cereal, *Dev. Psychobiol.*, 35, 197, 1999.
2. Gerrish, C.J. and Mannella, J.A., Flavor variety enhances food acceptance in formula-fed infants, *Am. J. Clin. Nutr.*, 73, 1080, 2001.
3. Mennella, J.A. and Beauchamp, G.K., Mothers' milk enhances the acceptance of cereal during weaning, *Pediatr. Res.*, 41, 188, 1997.
4. Birch, L.L. and Fisher, J.O., Development of eating behaviors among children and adolescents, *Pediatrics*, 101, 539, 1998.
5. Birch, L.L. and Marlin, D.W., I don't like it; I never tried it: effects of exposure to food on two-year-old children's food preferences, *Appetite*, 4, 353, 1982a.
6. Birch, L.L. et al., Effects of instrumental eating on children's food preferences, *Appetite*, 3, 125, 1982b.
7. Birch, L.L. et al., Clean up your plate: effects of child feeding practices on the conditioning of meal size, *Learn. Motiv.*, 18, 301, 1987.
8. Sullivan, S. and Birch., L., Pass the sugar; pass the salt: experience dictates preference, *Dev. Psychol.*, 26, 546, 1990.
9. Sullivan, S.A. and Birch, L.L., Infant dietary experience and acceptance of solid food, *Pediatrics*, 93, 271, 1994.

10. Birch, L.L., Marlin, D.W., and Rotter, J., Eating as the "means" activity in a contingency: effects on young children's food preference, *Child Dev.*, 55, 432, 1984.
11. Newman, J. and Taylor, A., Effect of a means: end contingency on young children's food preferences, *J. Exp. Child Psychol.*, 64, 200, 1992.
12. Hertzler, A.A., Children's food patterns — a review. II family and group behavior, *J. Am. Diet. Assoc.*, 83, 555, 1983.
13. Eppright, E.S. et al., Dietary study methods, V: some problems in collecting dietary information about groups of children, *J. Am. Diet. Assoc.*, 28, 43, 1952.
14. Stanek, K., Abbott, D., and Cramer, S., Diet quality and the eating environment of preschool children, *J. Am. Diet. Assoc.*, 90, 1582, 1990.
15. Birch, L.L., Zimmerman, S., and Hind, H., The influences of social-affective context on preschool children's food preferences, *Child Dev.*, 51, 856, 1980.
16. Birch, L.L., Dimensions of preschool children's food preferences, *J. Nutr. Educ.*, 11, 77, 1979a.
17. Birch, L.L., Preschool children's food preferences and consumptions patterns, *J. Nutr. Educ.*, 11, 189, 1987b.
18. Domel, S.B. et al., Measuring fruit and vegetable preferences among 4th and 5th grade students, *Prev. Med.*, 22, 866, 1993.
19. Fisher, J.A. and Birch, L.L., Three-to 5-year-old children's fat preferences and fat consumption are related to parental adiposity, *JADA*, 95, 759, 1995.
20. Domel, S.B. et al., Psychosocial predictors of fruit and vegetable consumption among elementary school children, *Health Educ. Res.*, 11, 299, 1996.
21. Birch, L.L. et al., What kind of exposure reduces children's food neophobia?, *Appetite*, 26, 546, 1990.
22. Birch, L.L. et al., The variability of young children's energy intake, *N. Engl. J. Med.*, 324, 232, 1991.
23. Birch, L.L. et al., Effects of a non-energy fat substitute on children's energy and macronutrient intake, *Am. J. Clin. Nutr.*, 58, 326, 1993.
24. Satter, E.M., The feeding relationship, *J. Am. Diet. Assoc.*, 86, 352, 1986.
25. Satter, E.M., Internal regulation and the evaluation of normal growth as a basis for prevention of obesity in children, *J. Am. Diet. Assoc.*, 96, 860, 1996.
26. Van Horn, L.V. et al., The Dietary Intervention Study in Children (DISC): dietary assessment methods for 8–10-year-olds, *JADA*, 93, 1396, 1993.
27. Meredith, A. et al., How well do school children recall what they have eaten?, *J. Am. Diet. Assoc.*, 27, 749, 1951.
28. Eppright, E.S. et al., Nutrition of infants and preschool children in the north central region of the United States of America, *World Rev. Nutr. Diet.*, 14, 269, 1972.
29. Emmons, L. and Hayes, M., Accuracy of 24-hr recalls of young children, *J. Am. Diet. Assoc.*, 62, 409, 1973.
30. Persson, L.A. and Carlgren, G., Measuring children's diets: evaluation of dietary assessment techniques in infancy and childhood, *Int. Epidemiol.*, 13, 506, 1984.
31. Baranowski, T. et al., The accuracy of children's self reports of diet: family health project, *J. Am. Diet. Assoc.*, 86, 1381, 1986.
32. Eck, L.H., Klesges, R.C., and Hanson, C.L., Recall of a child's intake from one meal: are parents accurate?, *J. Am. Diet. Assoc.*, 89, 784, 1989.

33. Treiber, F. et al., Dietary assessment instruments for preschool children: reliability of parental responses to the 24-hour recall and food frequency questionnaire, *J. Am. Diet. Assoc.*, 90, 814, 1990.
34. Van Horn, L. et al., Dietary assessment in children using electronic methods: telephones and tape recorders, *J. Am. Diet. Assoc.*, 90, 412, 1990.
35. Jaffe, A., Radius, S., and Gall, M., Health counseling for adolescents: what they want, what they get and who gives it, *Pediatrics*, 82, 481, 1988.

6

MOTIVATIONAL INTERVIEWING FOR CHILDREN AND ADOLESCENTS: STAGE 2

6.1 CHANGING DIETARY HABITS IN ADOLESCENTS

Resnicow reviews studies where motivational interviewing is the basic theoretical construct used to modify weight in children or adolescents [1]. Several studies are described below, ending with the Dietary Intervention Study in Children (DISC), where motivational interviewing was used as a way to increase adherence to a modified fat dietary pattern in children who had elevated LDL-cholesterol. An example of motivational interviewing used in this study is presented.

This first study, Healthy Lifestyles Pilot Study, is a 6-month intervention using motivational interviewing focused on children between the ages of 3 and 7 [2]. This study occurred in primary care pediatric settings with the aim of studying the efficacy and feasibility of the combination of pediatrician and dietitian MI counseling to prevent obesity in children. The study began with 15 practices randomly assigned to 1 of 3 conditions (5 practices per condition): (1) control, (2) minimal intervention, or (3) intensive intervention. Children's parents in the control arm of the study were given two printed sheets with tips on safety. In the minimal intervention, the pediatrician delivered a single brief MI counseling session 1 month from baseline. In the intensive intervention, the dietitian and pediatrician delivered two MI counseling sessions at 1 and 3 months from baseline. At 6 months there was a decrease of 0.4, 1.7, and 3.1 BMI percentile points in the control, minimal, and intensive intervention groups, respectively.

The Go Girls study included African American adolescent girls who were overweight. The intervention was a church-based nutrition and physical activity program [3]. The study did not include a control group. High- and moderate-intensity intervention groups were compared. For both interventions, group sessions included preparation and tasting of healthy foods, a behavioral activity and 30 minutes of physical activity. Those girls in the moderate intensity group received this culturally tailored intervention for 6 sessions with the high-intensity group receiving 20 to 26 sessions. Additionally, the high-intensity group received 4 to 6 motivational interviewing telephone counseling calls. Although the high-intensity group compared to the moderate-intensity group had a net decrease of 0.5 BMI units (p = 0.20), the study results were not statistically significant.

Channon and her colleagues used motivational interviewing with 22 adolescents (14 to 18 years of age) [4]. In a 6-month period, those teens received 4.7 sessions on average. The results in this study were statistically significant with reductions in HbA1c from 10.8% at baseline to 10.0% at 6-month follow-up.

In a small study involving only 6 teens between the ages of 13 and 16, Knight and colleagues administered an MI-based group intervention in 6 weekly 1-hour sessions [5]. The teens had been diagnosed with uncontrolled type I diabetes, with the goal of the study being to alter their attitude toward the disease. Therefore, changes in physiologic and behavioral outcomes were not assessed. The intervention used MI as a counseling strategy with "externalizing conversations" as a part of the theoretical basis for the intervention participants. The experimental group was compared to a "usual care" control group (n = 14). At 6 months, adolescents in the group MI intervention, compared with controls, displayed positive changes in their perception of diabetes. This included increased feelings of control as they dealt with the daily tasks of managing their disease.

The DISC study was a randomized, multicenter controlled trial with the focus on decreasing LDL-cholesterol in children. DISC began by focusing on group-based dietary intervention. In the initial stages of the study, this type of education-based intervention worked well. As the study progressed, dietary adherence began to decrease. To solve this problem, more focused interventions using MI strategies based on the transtheoretical model were initiated [6]. This model includes tailored approaches. First, detailed individual feedback looking at compliance over time is assessed by the adolescent. Second, the adolescent is asked to evaluate his or her adherence to diet by selecting a degree of adherence between

1 and 12 on a ruler. With this information, the nutrition counselor assigns a category:

1. Ready to change
2. Not ready to change
3. Unsure of readiness to change

This method to achieve behavior change is especially appropriate for adolescents [7–12]. Its use in DISC showed that it could be beneficial. Eating behaviors to reduce intakes of total fat and, specifically, saturated fat were successfully modified [13]. Preliminary data from this study showed that the mean proportion of calories from total fat decreased from 27.7 to 25.6% ($p < 0.001$) with a decrease of calories from saturated fat going from 9.5 to 8.6% ($p < 0.001$). In addition, consumption of dietary cholesterol decreased from 182.8 to 157.3 mg/1000 kcal ($p < 0.003$). Gender differences were not observed. Using a ruler to identify most-ready-to-change as 12, with 1 as least-ready-to-change, participants' readiness-to-change score increased by approximately 1 point ($p < 0.001$). Action plans were made by 94% of the participants and successfully implemented by 89% [13].

Initially, the assessment involves determining the readiness-to-change level (ready, unsure, not ready). Using a ruler or a scale concept ask, "On a scale of 1 to 12, how ready are you to make new changes to eat less fat? (1 = not ready to change; 12 = very ready to change)."

Adolescents might move from one readiness-to-change category to another during an interview. This means that the nutrition counselor must be ready to move back and forth between category-specific strategies. Clues that an adolescent has changed the readiness-to-change category might be confusion, detachment, or resistance during discussions. This is the nutrition counselor's prompt to reassess readiness-to-change, tailoring to a different stage of change if necessary.

A crucial point to remember is that every counseling session does not have to end with adolescent agreement. A decision to think about change is a successful conclusion to a motivational interviewing session.

6.2 NOT-READY-TO-CHANGE COUNSELING SESSION

The not-ready-to-change intervention involves the following three goals:

1. Facilitate the adolescent's ability to consider change
2. Reduce the adolescent's resistance to the change
3. Identify steps to change that are tailored to the individual adolescent's needs

There are several communication skills that will help in achieving these goals:

Open-ended questions: An open-ended question requires more than a "yes" or "no" answer. It is answered by explaining or discussing. For example:

"Tell me about how your dietary change experiences are going."
"What do you like about the changes you have made so far in your diet? What problems are connected with making these changes?"

Reflective listening: Listening in a reflective way involves identifying feelings that surface during a description of problems that result from changing eating habits. This type of listening is more than just paraphrasing words an adolescent has spoken. Reflective listening includes a guess at what the adolescent feels and is restated as a statement not a question. This skill communicates what the adolescent feels and is paraphrased as a statement. This allows the nutrition counselor to more fully understand true adolescent feelings. For example:

Adolescent: "I really want to do well with my diet, but my friends seem to entice me to eat out, and their selection of places is not a good fit for my new eating pattern."
Caregiver: "You feel frustrated because you really want to change your eating habits but at the same time you want to be spontaneous with friends."

Affirming: Adolescents so often feel at odds with authority figures and see adults as less than supportive. The skill of affirmation involves the counselor telling the adolescent that he or she, as an adult, understands and is with him or her in difficult times when diet change is not easy. Another important concept is normalization, where the caregiver tells the adolescent that he or she is perfectly within reason and that it is very normal to have such reactions and feelings. For example:

"I know that it is difficult for you to talk with me about this problem you are having with dietary change, but thank you for making this effort."
"You have had an incredible schedule with sports, academics, and being the lead in your school play. I feel that you have done extremely well given your circumstances."
"Many of the teens I talk with express the same problems. I can understand why you are having difficulty."

Summarizing: To keep an adolescent's attention, summarizing key concepts discussed during the session assures that the counselor understands issues that are often complex. A summarizing statement will help an adolescent only if it is simple and straightforward. In the case of teens, often the summary might involve descriptions of negative feelings.

Eliciting self-motivational statements: The four communication skills described above are important to this final strategy, eliciting self-motivational statements. The goals of these statements to facilitate the adolescent's realization are threefold:

1. That a problem exists; for example:
   ■ "I know that your friends are always eating out after school, what specifically makes this a problem for you?"
   ■ "Tell me, from your point of view as a teen, in what ways has following your diet been a problem?"
2. That concern exists about it; for example:
   ■ "When you give in to your teenage friends and eat high-fat foods, how do you feel?"
   ■ "Describe your concerns when you just can't eat what you would like to eat after a basketball game."
   ■ "What are your concerns if you don't make a change in the foods you are eating?"
3. That in the future, positive steps can be taken to correct the problem; for example:
   ■ "If you could eat in a way that is healthy all the time, what would need to be different for you?"
   ■ "What do you see as advantages to making dietary changes that reduce saturated fat?"
   ■ "If you decided to make a change in late night snacking while you study, what would need to happen?"
   ■ "You have done many things in sports that require devotion and dedication. What makes you think that if you decided to make a dietary change you could do it?"
   ■ "What encourages you that you can change if you want to?"
   ■ "If you decided to change, what strategies would help you maintain that change?"

It is important to be tentative when approaching a teen about problem eating behaviors: "Would you be willing to continue our discussion and talk about the possibility of change?"

In order to allow time for a thoughtful discussion around eating habits, ask open-ended questions or command statements.

"Tell me why you picked _____ on the ruler."

"What would need to happen for you to move from a 3 to a 12 on the ruler? What might I do to help you get there?"

Teens are very responsive to helping, attentive adults. To demonstrate this helping attitude, summarize statements about (1) past progress, (2) difficulties, (3) reasons for change, and (4) what would help in moving forward. This summarization will allow the teen to rethink the rationale for change.

Counselors often strive for goal-setting behaviors in adolescents. In this stage of change, forcing goal-setting behaviors will only cause feelings of defeat for both the teen and counselor:

"I can understand why this is a difficult time for you to make changes in your eating habits. Just being able to state the problems you are having is a very positive step forward. Things do change in our lives, especially in moving from teenage to adult years. When you are ready to discuss changes, I am always available. Based on decisions you have made in the past, I know you will come back to me when the time is right."

A crucial topic to cover prior to ending the session is the confidence and hope you have in the teen's ability to make changes. Finally, arrange for a follow-up contact.

As nutrition counselors, dealing with teens can be frustrating. Avoid the urge to push, coax, persuade, confront, or direct. Moving from one stage of change to another for a teen might not occur in the office setting. Do *not* expect a teen to commit to major changes during a visit. In fact, in this stage it might mean that the teen is merely trying to please you. In summary, strive for an open, caring environment that allows the teen to feel in control of making changes related to eating habits.

6.3 UNSURE-ABOUT-CHANGE COUNSELING SESSIONS

The goal in this stage is to build readiness to change, so that major steps can be taken to alter dietary adherence. In this stage, teens are ambivalent about making a change in their eating habits. To explore this ambivalence the nutrition counselor should ask the teen to list the positive and negative aspects of making changes in eating habits. For example:

"Tell me some of the things you like about old higher-saturated-fat eating habits."

"What are some of the good things about changing your eating habits?"

The nutrition counselor's goal is to help the teen consider change. This will occur by guiding the teen to a discussion about what life might be like after a change. By anticipating the advantages and disadvantages of modifying eating habits, the teen has the chance to see both sides of the issue of dietary change. To generate a discussion with the teen, the caregiver might begin with, "I can see why you're not totally sure of making new or additional changes in the way you eat. Imagine that you decided to make a change. What could that be like and what specifically would you want to do?" Finally, the nutrition counselor summarizes the positive and negative characteristics of making a change and includes statements that describe potential plans for change.

It is important to negotiate change with the teen. Initially, set broad goals with specific goals to follow. "How would you like things to be different?" and "What do you want to change?"

The teen might be asked to list strategies for dietary change. If one does not work, others might. Then the teen is asked to formulate a plan and write it down. To conclude the session, ask, "What do you plan to do between now and the next visit?"

The final statement should give the teen courage to make decisions. "I will not force you into achieving your goals. You have said that you are unsure. Take your time and know that I am always available to help you."

6.4 READY-TO-CHANGE COUNSELING SESSIONS

Meeting the goal of this stage requires collaboration with the teen to set a plan for action. The nutrition counselor should facilitate this plan by providing tools to use in meeting goals.

Questioning around change involves helping the teen confirm and rationalize the decision to make a change. Using the ruler again ask, "Why did you choose a 3 instead of a 1 or a 12? Give me some ideas for why you think you are ready to change."

Focus on helping the teen identify a first step in making a change. "What specifically could you do at school to make a change in your eating habits? Is this a truly workable plan? How will things be different for you if you make these changes?"

Goal setting becomes very important in this stage. Often teens will want to push ahead too fast. Realistic and achievable short-term goals are important. "Let's do things gradually. What is a short-term goal that you know is positioned for success?"

Following the setting of a short-term achievable goal, the patient might map out the specifics of how to be successful. Identify barriers to success. Doing this early will allow the teen to formulate ideas to overcome barriers or avoid them. Identify supportive family and friends to call on when eating healthful foods becomes a problem. Help the teen identify when a plan is successful. Ask the teen to write the plan down to document it for future discussions.

Close the session by giving encouraging comments and praising the teen for identifying the specifics of the plan. Emphasize that he or she is the expert on his or her own behavior. "You have come so far. It's clear that you are an expert on what is good for you. Keep in mind that change is gradual. If this plan doesn't work, there are others to try."

As with all of the stages, avoid giving advice. It is critical that the teen be allowed to express ideas for goals that will achieve the greatest success. Allow the teen to feel in control of changing eating behaviors. "I could give you a variety of goals, but what do you think will work best for you?"

In summary, changing eating habits for teens can be a highly successful endeavor. Keys to positive change include allowing the teen to make decisions about how to alter eating habits, proceeding gradually with change, and emphasizing that goal setting should depend on a teen's specific category of readiness to change. Only set specific goals when the teen is ready to change.

REFERENCES

1. Resnicow, K., Motivational interviewing: application to pediatric obesity — conceptual issues and evidence review, *J. Am. Diet. Assoc.*, in press.
2. Wasserman, R., Slora, E., and Bocian, A. et al., Pediatric research in office settings (PROS): a national practice-based research network to improve children's health care, *Pediatrics*, 102, 1350, 1998.
3. Resnicow, K., Taylor, R., and Baskin, M., Results of Go Girls: a nutrition and physical activity intervention for overweight African American adolescent females conducted through black churches, *Obes. Res.* 13, 1739, 2005.
4. Channon, S., Smith, V.J., and Gregory, J.W., A pilot study of motivational interviewing in adolescents with diabetes, *Arch. Dis. Child.*, 88, 680, 2003.
5. Knight, K.M., Bundy, C., and Morris, R. et al., The effects of group motivational interviewing and externalizing conversations for adolescents with type-1 diabetes, *Psych., Health Med.*, 8, 149, 2003.
6. Prochaska, J. and DiClemente, C., Transtheoretical therapy: toward a more integrative model of change, *Psychotherapy: Theory, Research and Practice,* 19, 276, 1982.
7. Jaffe, A., Radius, S., and Gall, M., Health counseling for adolescents: what they want, what they get and who gives it, *Pediatrics,* 82, 481, 1988.
8. Werch, C.H. and DiClemente, C.C., A multi-component stage model for matching drug prevention strategies and messages to youth stage of use, *Health Educ. Res.,* 9, 37, 1994.
9. Rollnick, S. and Morgan, M., Motivational interviewing: increasing readiness to change, in *Psychotherapy and Substance Abuse. A Practitioner's Handbook,* Washton, A.M., Ed., New York: Guilford Press, 1991, 179–191.

10. Grimley, D. et al., Contraception and condom use adoption and maintenance: a stage paradigm approach, *Health Educ. Q.,* 22, 20, 1995.
11. Christopher, J., Nangle, D., and Hansen, D., Social skills interventions with adolescents, *Behav. Modif.,* 17, 314, 1994.
12. Tober, G., Motivational interviewing with young people, in *Motivational Interviewing*, Miller, W.R. and Rollnick, S., Eds., New York: Guilford Press, 1991, 248–259.
13. Berg-Smith, S.M. et al., For the Dietary Intervention Study in Children (DISC) Research Group, brief motivational intervention to improve dietary adherence in adolescents, *Health Educ. Res.,* 14, 399, 1999.

7

MOTIVATIONAL INTERVIEWING FOR ADULTS AND THE ELDERLY: STAGE 3

Motivational interviewing has been used in many studies including adult populations. Resnicow reviews studies where motivational interviewing has been used to modify diet and physical activity behaviors [1]. Several studies are described below ending with the Women's Health Initiative (WHI) study where motivational interviewing was used as a way to increase adherence to a low-fat dietary pattern. An example of motivational interviewing used in this study is presented.

The first study is a pilot where Smith and colleagues studied 22 overweight women (41% African American) with type 2 diabetes [2]. The study included two types of intervention; one was a 16-week behavioral weight control group format and the other the same intervention with 16 women receiving the addition of three individual MI sessions. The first MI session was delivered at baseline before group treatment began, with two sessions delivered at mid-treatment. The MI sessions focused on individualized feedback on blood glucose control. Subjects were counseled to review data that showed a discrepancy between current status and desired goals. A post-test at 4 months showed that the women who received the MI had significantly better glycemic control, were more consistent in monitoring their blood glucose, and attended more sessions than those in the comparison group.

Mhurchu, with coinvestigators, randomly assigned 121 patients with hyperlipidemia to receive either three MI sessions or a standard dietary intervention, both delivered by a dietitian [3]. The study looked at differences in diet and BMI at 3 months and found no statistically significant results comparing the two groups. Tape recordings of the two types of interventions revealed that more reflective listening, a hallmark of MI, occurred in the MI sessions with more advice-giving in the standard intervention. Because 80% of the sample was making dietary changes at baseline (i.e., they were in an advanced stage of change), significant differences in groups might have been difficult to achieve.

Woollard and coworkers randomly assigned 166 hypertensive patients to one of three groups: (1) high intensity MI (six 45-minute sessions every 4th week), (2) low intensity MI (a single face-to-face session plus five brief telephone contacts), or (3) a control group [4]. There were no significant differences between the two MI groups noted at the 18-month follow-up. However, the high intensity MI group had significantly reduced their weight and blood pressure relative to controls, whereas the low intensity MI group significantly decreased their alcohol and salt intake relative to controls.

In a group of 523 adults, Harland and investigators randomly assigned the group to four intervention groups [5]: two groups received a single 40-minute MI session and two received six 40-minute MI sessions delivered over 12 weeks, with half of the participants receiving vouchers for free aerobics classes. There was also a control group that received neither MI nor vouchers. At 12 weeks, self-reported physical activity improved in the four combined intervention groups relative to the controls (38% improved vs. 16%).

Resnicow and his colleagues in the Eat for Life (EFL) trial designed a multicomponent intervention to increase fruit and vegetable consumption among African American adults [6]. Fourteen churches were randomly assigned to one of three treatment conditions: (1) control, (2) "culturally-tailored self-help" (SH) intervention with one telephone call used to increase use of SH intervention materials, and (3) SH intervention, one cue call, and three MI counseling calls. Self-reported fruit and vegetable consumption at 1 year was significantly greater in the MI group than the control and SH groups.

Resnicow and colleagues also participated in the Body and Soul project. In this study, the intervention was constructed from two prior church-based behavior change programs, Black Churches United for Better Health and Eat for Life [7]. The intervention included church-wide activities, distribution of self-help materials, and peer counseling. In Eat for Life, the MI was delivered by trained dietitians; in Body and Soul, MI was facilitated by trained lay church members, referred to as volunteer advisors. A total of 1022 individuals were recruited from the 15 churches (8 intervention and 7 control) participating in the study with 854 (84%) retained for 6-month follow-up. In the final visit, participants in the intervention group reported significantly greater consumption of fruits and vegetables than those in the control group.

The final adult intervention is the Healthy Body Healthy Spirit study [8]. The primary aim of the study was to increase fruit and vegetable consumption and physical activity among a socioeconomically diverse sample of African Americans. The fruit and vegetable intervention was an adaptation from the Eat for Life trial. Sixteen churches were randomly assigned to three intervention conditions. At baseline, a total of 1056 individuals were recruited across the 16 churches, of which 906 (86%) were assessed at 1 year. Group 1 received standard educational materials; Group 2 received culturally targeted self-help nutrition and physical activity materials; and Group 3 received the same intervention as Group 2, plus four telephone counseling calls (at weeks 4, 12, 26, and 40), based on MI delivered over the course of 1 year.

The primary outcomes were self-reported fruit and vegetable intake and minutes of physical activity. At 1 year, Groups 2 and 3 showed significant changes in both fruit and vegetable consumption and physical activity. Changes were somewhat larger for fruit and vegetable intake vs. the physical activity with a clear positive effect attributed to the MI intervention.

With the exception of the study completed by Mhurchu and colleagues, each study reviewed above showed a significant effect favoring the MI group on at least one main outcome. Below is a brief review of motivational interviewing as it was used in the WHI to enhance adherence to a low-fat dietary eating style.

To maintain dietary adherence in WHI, novel counseling programs were used in the Diet Modification (DM) arm of the study [9]. One ancillary study implemented after the parent WHI study began was designed to evaluate the efficacy of an intensive intervention program (IIP) based on MI to increase dietary adherence in WHI women. The study included a subset of 3 out of the 40 clinical centers involved in WHI. Women from these three centers were randomly assigned to either the intervention or control group. Those women in the intervention group received three individual MI contacts from a nutrition counselor, plus the usual WHI Dietary Intervention in small groups.

The usual WHI Dietary Intervention included sessions held once every 3 months. The sessions focused on food demonstrations, and discussions around healthy foods and the nutrients they provide. Discussions also occurred with women relating their successes and failures. The small groups were a support for women having difficulties with dietary adherence and a reaffirmation of women doing well. Women assigned to the control group received the usual WHI Dietary Intervention without the three additional motivational interviewing contacts.

For the ancillary study, data used to compare the MI intervention and control groups were based on the percent of energy from fat using a food frequency questionnaire. Comparisons were made between the ancillary study baseline and follow-up 1 year later in the two study groups. The change in percent of calories from fat comparing baseline and year 1 was −1.2% for the IIP program participants. In IIP control participants, the percent of calories from fat went up by 1.4%. The result was an overall difference between the two groups of 2.6% ($p < 0.001$). Those participants in the ancillary study who had the largest overall change in percent of calories from fat were those with the highest baseline fat intake.

In the IIP study each MI contact consisted of three steps: (1) assessment, (2) intervention, and (3) future directions. During assessment, using a series of yes/no questions, participants were assigned to one of three intervention phases: Phase 1 included those who were not ready to make changes in their diet, Phase 2 included those unsure of making dietary changes, and Phase 3 included those who were ready to change. The assessment step was designed to help participants see discrepancies between actual dietary adherence and their own perceptions of adherence, using data describing fat grams eaten each day from self-monitoring forms. Initially nutrition counselors showed participants a graph indicating the distance between their current progress and the overall WHI study goals. This data led to a discussion of the participant's positive changes in attaining her personal fat gram goal, her interest in making further changes, and barriers to success in dietary modification.

7.1 INTERVENTION PHASE 1 (NOT READY TO CHANGE)

In this phase the nutrition counselor is focused on helping the participant identify the need for change, reduce resistance including barriers to change, and, finally, increase interest in the possibility of making a dietary change. The nutrition counselor encourages the participant to discuss the possible reasons for change. The nutrition counselor asks a question such as: "What would need to be different to move forward and what will prevent that forward move?"

The following is a list of sample questions that might encourage change in nutrition lifestyle:

Open-ended questions: "If you were to project out for the next year, what do you think your dietary adherence would look like?" (A graph of adherence to diet over time might be used here.)
"Do you have any reasons why you wouldn't want to lower your fat grams any further?"
"Where does this leave you now?"

Emphasizing choice: "The decision is up to you. It is okay to go home and think about this for a while. I will always be here to help whenever you wish to talk again."

7.2 INTERVENTION PHASE 2 (UNSURE ABOUT CHANGE)

In this phase, building readiness to change is the key. The participant is asked to list positive and negative aspects of changing nutrition lifestyle. The question that might be asked is: "What are the resulting difficulties and advantages of making changes in your diet?" The goal is for the participant to identify future dietary plans, with the topic of change being initially posed by the participant. In this phase it is important to avoid assuming that a participant is ready to change when that might not be true.

Examples of questions and phrases that might be used to build readiness for change in dietary lifestyle include the following: Emphasize that the change is their choice: "But the decision is really yours." Or "It will be up to you whether you decide to make a change."

Affirming by referring to past successes can be helpful in moving toward change: "I am confident, having watched your track record and what you've been able to do in the past that you can be successful." Or "I have a lot of confidence in you."

7.3 INTERVENTION PHASE 3 (READY TO CHANGE)

The role of the nutrition counselor in this phase is to facilitate each participant's work on planning dietary change. It is critical in this phase that the idea for change comes from the participant. The initial question is: "What would you like to change in your diet?" Or "What are some strategies that you might use if the changes you hope to make do not work out for you?"

Then, set realistic and achievable short-term goals, followed by an action plan developed by the participant. To end the session use of affirming statements similar to the following will be of value in assuring the possibility of success:

"I am really confident in your abilities to make the changes we discussed today."

"Remember that you are the expert in deciding what will work for you. However, if you ever need to talk about problems you are having I am always here."

"Keep in mind that you have many options. If the goals you have set now do not work, there are a number of directions to go in to ensure that you can meet the goals."

Following this ancillary study, nutrition counselors began using MI with all of the WHI participants in the parent study, not just the few in the ancillary study. For those WHI parent study women, a recent article suggests that MI combined with group counseling was effective in weight loss and maintenance of that loss [10]. Data from the WHI DM arm of the study showed that a comparison of the dietary intervention group with the women in the control group following their usual American diet lost weight in the first year and maintained that loss after an average of 7.5 years of follow-up (1.9 kg, $p < 0.001$ at year 1 and 0.4 kg, $p = 0.01$ at 7.5 years). Also of importance was the result that the intervention group did not exhibit a tendency toward weight gain throughout this 7.5-year period. This is interesting in that the dietary counseling in the WHI was not aimed at decreasing calories. Also, the group sessions were not focused on weight loss. In fact, the consent form that WHI women were required to sign upon entry into the study emphasized the fact that this was not a study designed for weight loss. The major aim of the DM arm of the study was based on decreasing total fat and increasing fruits, vegetables, and all types of grains. The study also looked at all women combined from both the intervention and control groups of the WHI parent study. In those women who were able to decrease their percent of energy from fat, regardless of which group they were in, weight loss was greatest. A similar but lesser trend was observed in those women who were able to increase their servings of fruits and vegetables. Increases in intake of fiber also resulted in a nonsignificant trend toward weight loss. Again, increases in fiber were not a major focus of the DM intervention.

For the many women concerned about their weight, reductions in fat might, but do not necessarily always, decrease calories substantially. A panel of nutritionists serving on the National Institutes of Health, Obesity Education Initiative [11] designed menus to consider both the type and quantity of fat along with level of calories. Menus were designed with ethnicity in mind. An exchange list to allow for substitutions in menu selections was also created. In addition to the publication [12], the menus are available on the Internet at www.nhlbi.nih.gov/guidelines/obesity/practgde.htm.

7.4 SUMMARY

In summary, MI is a positive method of facilitating changes in diet with moderate decreases in weight loss. It promotes assessment of patients' readiness for dietary change and provides for stage-based guidance in adopting long-term nutrition lifestyle changes to reduce risk for chronic disease.

REFERENCES

1. Resnicow, K., Motivational interviewing: application to pediatric obesity — conceptual issues and evidence review, *J. Am. Diet. Assoc.,* in press.
2. Smith, D., Heckemeyer, D., Kratt, P., and Mason, D., Motivational interviewing to improve adherence to a behavioral weight-control program for older obese women with NIDDM, *Diabetes Care,* 20, 52, 1997.
3. Mhurchu, C.N., Margetts, B.M., and Speller, V., Randomized clinical trial comparing the effectiveness of two dietary interventions for patients with hyperlipidaemia, *Clinical Science,* 95, 479, 1998.
4. Woollard, J., Beilin, L., Lord, T., Puddey, I., MacAdam, D., and Rouse, I., A controlled trial of nurse counseling on lifestyle change for hypertensives treated in general practice: preliminary results, *Clinical & Experimental Pharmacology & Physiology,* 22, 466, 1995.
5. Harland, J., White, M., Drinkwater, C., Chinn, D., Farr, L., and Howel, D., The Newcastle exercise project: a randomized controlled trial of methods to promote physical activity in primary care, *British Med. J.,* 319, 828, 1999.
6. Resnicow, K., Jackson, A., Wang, T., Dudley, W., and Baranowski, T., A motivational interviewing intervention to increase fruit and vegetable intake through black churches: results of the Eat for Life Trial, *Am. J. Public Health,* 91, 1686, 2001.
7. Resnicow, K., Campbell, M.K., and Carr, C. et al., Body and soul A dietary intervention conducted through African-American churches, *Am. J. Preventive Med.,* 27, 97, 2004.
8. Resnicow, K., Jackson, A., and Blissett, D. et al., Results of the Healthy Body Healthy Spirit Trial, *Health Psychol.,* 24, 339, 2005.
9. Bowen, D., Ehret, C., Pedersen, M., Snetselaar, L., Johnson, M., Tinker, L., Hollinger, D., Lichty, I., Bland, K., Sivertsen, D., Ocken, D., Staats, L., and Beedoe, J.W., Results of an adjunct dietary intervention program in the Women's Health Initiative, *J. Am. Diet Assoc.,* 102, 1631–1637, 2002.
10. Howard, B.V., Manson, J.E., Stefanick, M.L., Beresford, S.A., Frank, G., Jones, B., Rodabough, R.J., Snetselaar, L., Thomson, C., Tinker, L., Vitolins, M., and Prentice, R., Low-fat dietary pattern and weight change over 7 years — the Women's Health Initiative Dietary Modification Trial, *JAMA,* 295, 39, 2006.
11. Expert Panel, Clinical Guidelines on the Identification, Evaluation, and Treatment of Overweight and Obesity in Adults, National Heart, Lung, and Blood Institute in cooperation with the National Institute of Diabetes and Digestive and Kidney Diseases, NIH Publication No. 98-4083, September, 1998, National Institutes of Health.
12. Expert Panel, The Practical Guide to the Identification, Evaluation, and Treatment of Overweight and Obesity in Adults, National Heart, Lung, and Blood Institute in cooperation with the National Institute of Diabetes and Digestive and Kidney Diseases, NIH Publication No. 00-4083, October, 2000, National Institutes of Health. Available at: www.nhlbi.nih.gov/guidelines/obesity/practgde.htm, accessed on March 18, 2004.

8

INNOVATIVE APPROACHES
TO MAINTAINING
HEALTHY BEHAVIORS

Clinicians have identified two problems with behavior change and its maintenance: time to provide the intervention in a clinical setting and the difficulties with achieving lifestyle change given the increasing prevalence of patients with multiple risk factors. Glasgow [1] references an article that indicates the delivery of preventive services recommended by the U.S. Preventive Services Task Force (USPSTF) [2] to an average number of patients. Calculations based on the services proscribed show that family physicians would need to spend 7.5 hours of every working day on prevention to meet the USPSTF recommendations [3]. The challenging complexity of changing many behaviors associated with multiple chronic illnesses makes it necessary to be creative in providing services. Many researchers are pointing to a combination of brief in-person counseling and interactive behavior change technology (IBCT).

IBCT is defined as a combination of computer-based tools and systems, including hardware and software, that allows for increased health behavior change without excess amounts of time provided by the clinician in person. Several examples include CD-ROM interventions using touch-screen kiosks that incorporate the stages of change theoretical framework proposed by Prochaska and DiClemente [4]; personal digital assistants (PDAs) or other handheld devices; electronic medical records or registries that include behavior change information; and interactive voice response (IVR) technologies [5].

Glasgow and others recommend the five A's model of counseling (assess, advise, agree, assist, and arrange follow-up) when using IBCT [1].

The five A's are sequential and dynamic, emphasizing behavior change over time. They include using assessment techniques to define baseline dietary and other health-related behaviors. Advising around those known baseline behaviors includes personally relevant ways to change health risk behaviors. Advising can take the form of the patient's pros and cons for doing specific healthy behaviors. Agreeing on behavior change goals is an important step in negotiating strategies to alter at-risk habits. The next step is to assist the patient in problem-solving strategies that eliminate barriers to change and maximize strengths to attain goals. Finally, the arrangement of follow-up support is negotiated to achieve and maintain behavior changes.

Apart from the clinician, even before the patient begins a clinic visit, IBCT can assist in identifying baseline information through the first of the five A's — assessment. A health risk assessment (HRA) through telephone, a Web site, or CD-ROM can be done prior to a face-to-face medical encounter. Research shows that HRAs are effective in reaching goals of behavior change when they occur with feedback and support [6–8]. Preprogrammed algorithms can be used to tailor responses to the patient. For example, a patient who indicates a diet rich in fruits and vegetables might get a very positive reinforcement statement. For the patient who eats only one serving of a fruit or vegetable each day suggestions on how to gradually incorporate additional servings will be given. Research using these IBCT-tailored messages is mostly positive [9–17]. Two researchers indicate minimal effectiveness using this strategy [18, 19]. Research is needed to determine the types of tailoring that are most effective.

When printed messages are tailored allowing individual characteristics to drive the development of materials, they are more likely to be used by a patient in making behavior changes [16–18, 20, 21]. IBCT will allow for feedback to patients by tailoring to each individual's goal achievement level. With this feedback it is possible to provide the patient with strategies to maximize achievement of new goals. Printouts can be generated from this technology, allowing the patient and nutrition counselor to discuss goal attainment. For example, "Mrs. Jones has set a goal of including two additional fruits or vegetables in her lunch bag as a beginning to increasing her intake to eventually achieve at least five servings of fruits and vegetables a day." This message will be delivered to the patient and the nutrition counselor using several IBCT modalities. For the patient, completing an HRA, feedback could come in the form of a printout or online. The same information could go to the medical team, including the nutrition counselor, through e-mail or an electronic medical record.

Glasgow describes a variety of ways to minimize face-to-face time by allowing upfront patient communication [1] Although the development of a Web site has initial costs, it allows the patient to come to a face-to-face visit more informed and, from some research, more satisfied with providers' services [20, 22, 23]. The Health Information Portability and Accountability Act (HIPPAA) Privacy Rule provides mandates to assure confidentiality online. Initial IBCT information that tells the patient about insurance, parking, transportation, and what might happen during a dietary counseling visit is an important time-saving strategy. Additionally, a Web site could list a variety of questions from which the patient could select and bring with him or her to a clinic visit. The Web site might link to other sites; for example, the American Dietetic Association is developing an evidence-based Web site that would provide updated information on diseases and the research relative to nutrition in treating and preventing them. Patients often go to Web sites that may be less than accurate. With this feature of linking, the nutrition counselor has more control over what the patient sees, and less misinformation will need to be discussed during an office visit.

Another innovative way to set the stage prior to an office visit is the use of IVR technology. Glasgow discusses a creative way of determining previsit expectations, questions, and goals [1]. An IVR computer-based telephone system will allow for calling, receiving calls, presenting information, and collecting data from patients. For a patient with several behavioral health risks, the time in a visit might be too short to allow for adequate discussion of questions that focus on patient concerns. With an IVR call before a visit, patients will have the ability to identify concerns or questions. The patient responses could be inserted into the medical record and would be available to the medical team, including the nutrition counselor at the time of the face-to-face appointment. Piette and colleagues have used this means of communicating with success in large healthcare systems [24, 25]. Again HIPPAA regulations must be followed to protect the patient's privacy.

IBCT is also a useful tool following a visit. This technology can be used to monitor large patient groups and identify individuals with health- or self-care problems [25]. Studies show that IVR technology can provide valid and reliable information about healthcare for sensitive health problems where difficulty adhering to self-care plans occurs [24, 26, 27]. Randomized trials show that IVR monitoring with follow-up by a clinician improves self-managed care, perceived health status, and physiologic outcomes among persons who have diabetes and are hypertensive [28, 29]. Other forms of IBCT, such as the Internet, allow patients to monitor and receive feedback on changes relative to their own health and progress toward negotiated self-managed action plans [30].

In general, technology might be the answer to help in routinely reaching individuals at risk for chronic disease. The technology described in this chapter can be key to assisting in behavior change efforts in all three age stages described in previous chapters.

REFERENCES

1. Glasgow, R.E. et al., Interactive behavior change technology: a partial solution to the competing demands of primary care, *Am. J. Prev. Med.*, 27, 80, 2004.
2. U.S. Preventive Services Task Force, *Guide to Clinical Preventive Services.* 2nd ed., Baltimore, MD: Williams and Wilkins, 1996.
3. Yarnell, K.S. et al., Primary care: is there enough time for prevention?, *Am. J. Public Health*, 93, 635, 2003.
4. Prochaska, J. and DiClemente, C., Transtheoretical therapy: toward a more integrative model of change, *Psychotherapy: Theory, Research and Practice*, 19, 276, 1982.
5. Dertouzos, M.L., *What Will Be: How the New World of Information Will Change Our Lives*, New York: Harper Edge Publishers, 1997.
6. Pronk, N.P. and O'Connor, P., Systems approach to population health improvement, *J. Ambulatory Care Manage.*, 20, 24, 1997.
7. Babor, T.F., Sciamanna, C.N., and Pronk, N., Assessing multiple risk behaviors in prim car: screening issues and related concepts, *Am. J. Prev. Med.*, 27, 42, 2004.
8. Kreuter, M.W. and Stretcher, V.J., Do tailored behavior change messages enhance the effectiveness of health risk appraisal? Results from a randomized trial, *Health Educ. Res.*, 11, 97, 1996.
9. Bental, D.S., Cawsey, A., and Jones, R., Patient information systems that tailor to the individual, *Patient Educ. Couns.*, 2, 171, 1999.
10. Campbell, M.K. et al., Improving dietary behavior: the effectiveness of tailored messages in primary care settings, *Am. J. Public Health*, 84, 783, 1994.
11. DeVries, H. and Brug, J., Computer-tailored interventions motivating people to adopt health promoting behaviors: introduction to a new approach, *Patient Educ. Couns.*, 36, 99, 1999.
12. Kreuter, M.W. and Stretcher, V.J., Changing inaccurate perceptions of health risk: results from a randomized trial, *Health Psychol.*, 14, 56, 1995.
13. Lipkus, I.M., Lyna, P.R., and Rimer, B.K., Using tailored interventions to enhance smoking cessation among African-Americans at a community health center, *Nicotine Tob. Res.*, 1, 77, 1999.
14. Marcus, B.H. et al., Evaluation of motivationally tailored vs. standard self-help physical activity interventions at the workplace, *Am. J. Health Promo.*, 12, 246, 1998.
15. Rakowski, W. et al., Increasing mammography among women aged 40–74 by use of a stage-matched, tailored intervention, *Am. J. Prev. Med.*, 27, 748, 1998.
16. Skinner, C.S., Strecher, V.J., and Hospers, H., Physicians' recommendations for mammography: do tailored messages make a difference?, *Am. J. Public Health*, 84, 43, 1994.
17. Brug, J., Campbell, M., and Van Assema, P., The application and impact of computer-generated personalized nutrition education: a review of the literature, *Patient Educ. Couns.*, 36, 145, 1999.
18. Kreuter, M. et al., *Tailoring Health Messages: Customizing Communication with Computer Technology*, Mahweh, NJ: Lawrence Erlbaum, 2000.
19. Ryan, G.L. et al., Examining the boundaries of tailoring: the utility of tailoring versus targeting mammography interventions for two distinct populations, *Health Educ. Res.*, 16, 555, 2001.

20. Tate, D.F., Wing, F.F., and Winett, R.A., Using Internet technology to deliver a behavioral weight loss program, *JAMA*, 285, 1172, 2001.
21. Strecher, V.J. et al., The effects of computer-tailored smoking cessation messages in family practice settings, *J. Fam. Pract.*, 39, 262, 1994.
22. Gustafson, D.H. et al., Consumers and evaluation of interactive health communication applications. The Science panel on Interactive Communication and Health, *Am. J. Prev. Med.*, 16, 23, 1999.
23. Gustafson, D.H. et al., Impact of a patient-centered, computer-based health information/support system, *Am. J. Prev. Med.*, 16, 1, 1999.
24. Piette, J.D. et al., Use of automated telephone disease management calls in an ethnically diverse sample of low-income patients with diabetes, *Diabetes Care*, 22, 1302, 1999.
25. Piette, J.D., Patient education via automated calls: a study of English and Spanish speakers with diabetes, *Am. J. Prev. Med.*, 17, 138, 2000.
26. Perrine, M.W. et al., Validation of daily self-reported alcohol consumption using interactive voice response (IVR) technology, *J. Stud. Alcohol*, 56, 487, 1995.
27. Kobak, K.A. et al., A computer-administered telephone interview to identify mental disorders, *JAMA*, 278, 905, 1997.
28. Piette, J.D. et al., The impact of automated calls with nurse follow-up on diabetes treatment outcomes in Veterans Affairs health care system, *Diabetes Care*, 24, 202, 2001.
29. Friedman, R.H. et al., A telecommunications system for monitoring and counseling patients with hypertension, *Am. J. Hypertens.*, 9, 285, 1996.
30. Feil, E.G. et al., Who participates in Internet-based self-management programs? A study among novice computer users in a primary care setting, *Diabetes Educ.*, 26, 806, 2000.

9

TAILORING TO
PATIENT NEEDS

Tailoring dietary counseling to each patient's situation is the key to long-term lifestyle change. The concept of change depends on how closely new behaviors match old habits. Without knowledge of baseline behaviors, we have no map with which to chart the course of lifestyle change. The concept of one size fitting all is a formula for disaster in dietary counseling. Tailoring can apply to a variety of counseling formats and can be used in individual counseling and in group settings.

9.1 IDENTIFYING YOUR PATIENT

Without a clear understanding of patient characteristics, the foundation of counseling for lifestyle change is flawed.

9.1.1 Gender

Understanding gender differences in counseling for lifestyle change means knowing the ways in which food affects behavior. For example, a woman might see food as a symbol of affection and a man might focus on the effect eating a certain type of food has on his performance in sports. Each sees food as important but has a different focus on its benefit.

Two NIH funded, randomized, controlled, clinical trials show a stark comparison of gender. The Lipid Research Clinic Studies, in particular the Coronary Primary Prevention Trial (CPPT), an all-male study, and the Women's Health Initiative (WHI) Study, an all-female study, provide studies in gender differences. Few sessions in the CPPT were completed without both spouses or significant others present. It was very clear that the female partner in a traditional marriage was responsible for most of the cooking and played a huge role in the eating habits of the family. In nontraditional families cooperative relationships with food preparation were noted. In contrast, the WHI is an all-female study, where it is quite apparent that food preparation is solely the domain of the participant. Rarely are male spouses responsible for the majority of the food preparation. In nontraditional families, again the relationships relative to food preparation are often cooperative.

9.1.2 Age

This text has already classified persons according to age by focusing on three stages in lifestyle change. Working with different age groups requires an understanding of roles people play as they age. Often we stereotype age groups. For example, when we began the National Institutes of Health-funded WHI we had a stereotypical view of the focus elderly women would have on adherence to a low-fat dietary pattern. We thought that elderly retired women would use the diet as a focus and would be totally dedicated to the study through their latter years. What we found was that elderly women are often faced with monumental life events that affect their ability to adhere to dietary recommendations. They have spouses who are dying, placing them in a situation never before dealt with and forcing them to totally refocus their attention. They are required to become caregivers for children who run into difficulty and need both financial and emotional support. They become less structure-oriented and focus on spontaneity, with diet taking a lower priority than it may have taken in their younger years. They see life in terms of ending and the younger version of immortality is not a part of their vision. Also, life events can change their view of the importance of dietary adherence in a positive way. For example, a heart attack or finding out they have type 2 diabetes can lead to "teachable moments" that increase dietary adherence.

Young adults are often working very hard to raise families. They see diet as important for their children's health but also have time limitations. Those time limitations force them into a situation where eating to stay alive places everyone in a family on a time schedule. The enjoyment of purchasing, preparing, and calmly eating healthy foods becomes a secondary mission.

In homes where healthy eating is appreciated, often well-meaning parents will become so dogmatic in their desires to force a healthful lifestyle on their children that food aversions result, leaving children in a mode of constant food refusal. Research shows the importance of fostering healthy feeding practices in young children (see Chapter 5). Additional research shows us that disadvantaged populations can have the opposite problem, where too little modeling and structure results in poor eating habits [1–4]. These two divergent groups show us that culture is paramount in tailoring counseling strategies.

9.1.3 Ethnicity

Ethnicity pays a huge part in our ability to adequately tailor counseling strategies. As nutrition counselors, we might listen to Airhihenbuwa's words on the topic of communication with other cultures:

> The collective experience of a people (the culture) prepares them to deal with and sometimes subvert and transform oppressive conditions in ways unknown to the oppressor. Such experiences and their resultant wisdom transcend levels of income, age, and generation. We must never assume that because a group is economically poor its members are also cerebrally, philosophically, and practically poor, nor should we assume that wisdom in and of itself will overcome economic oppression. Programmatic efforts must, therefore, be directed toward synchronizing the philosophy of the people with their practices [5].

Kumanyika discusses the importance of ethnicity in the way we communicate with patients. She points to the fact that much of what we see in increased morbidity and mortality in persons of ethnicity might be a direct result of their lack of compliance to therapeutic regimens [6].

Initially it is important to define race and ethnicity as shown in Table 9.1. It is possible to separate race and ethnicity into categories, but Kumanyika cautions that as we work with dietary adherence, in concept they are intertwined, resulting in more complicated classification characteristics. It is often difficult to understand why adherence to diet might be different according to ethnicity because as studies are implemented, the process of recruitment focuses on selecting motivated groups within the ethnic populations. Kumanyika provides a summary of the research done, first looking at studies reporting differences in dietary adherence in ethnic groups (Table 9.2). Second, she describes those studies that have been specifically designed for effectiveness with ethnic populations (Table 9.3).

To summarize Tables 9.2 and 9.3, we find that, in general, ethnic populations tend to be less compliant than Caucasian populations. It must be noted that in many studies the original aim of the study was not to compare ethnic groups. In Table 9.2, Majonnier's research provided the only data showing that African American populations reported better dietary adherence than Caucasian study populations. All other studies

Table 9.1   Race Ethnicity Categories in the 1990 Census

Race	White
	Black or Negro
	Chinese
	Indian (Amer.)
	Japanese
	Filipino
	Asian Indian
	Korean
	Aleut
	Eskimo
	Hawaiian
	Vietnamese
	Guamanian
	Samoan
	Other Asian/Pacific Islander
	Other Race
Hispanic ethnicity	Mexican, Mexican Amer., Chicano
	Puerto Rican
	Cuban
	Other Spanish/Hispanic/Latino
	Not Spanish/Hispanic/Latino

Source: Pollard, K.M. and O'Hare, W.P., America's racial and ethnic minorities. Population Bulletin 54.3, Washington, D.C.: Population Reference Bureau, 1999.

showed that African American participants compared to Caucasian participants had more difficulties with dietary compliance.

Some studies have been designed for the purpose of identifying effectiveness in populations of ethnicity. Table 9.3 describes five studies where lifestyle change programs were specifically tailored to social cultural and contextual issues of ethnic populations. The studies in this table are different from Table 9.2 because they focus on the effectiveness of nutrition lifestyle change interventions within particular ethnic groups. Table 9.2 emphasizes relative effectiveness across ethnic groups.

Studies in Table 9.2 are important because they help in determining different expectations of dietary adherence success using cross-ethnic comparisons. These studies provide a longer time to achieve the dietary effect. Also, the studies point to the ethnic population's potential preference for certain strategies within the program that might be more positive in terms of dietary adherence success. They also allow us to discover problems that might result from using a general or more mainstream

Table 9.2 Studies Reporting Ethnic Differences in Direct or Indirect Measures of Dietary Adherence

Authors	Study Objective	Study Design	Findings
Mojonnier et al., 1980	Evaluation of nutrition education approaches in preparation for a trial of cardiovascular disease risk reduction	Participants (199 whites and 84 blacks) with hypercholesterolemia were randomly assigned to one of four teaching formats or to no education	Compared to whites, black participants had greater gains in knoledge at one month; at 6 to 9 month follow-up, black participants reported larger dietary changes and had greater reductions in serum cholesterol.
Kumanyika et al., 1991	Efficacy of weight reduction for the prevention of hypertension	Analyses of sex and race-specific results from two separate, randomized, controlled multi-center studies, involving men and women ages 25 to 49 (HPT) or 30 to 54 (TOHP) who were not using antihypertensive medications and had diastolic blood pressures between 80 and 89 mmHg at baseline; follow-up was 18 or 36 months	In both studies, mean overall weight change was less in blacks than whites; particularly among women.

Continued.

Table 9.2 Studies Reporting Ethnic Differences in Direct or Indirect Measures of Dietary Adherence (*Continued*)

Authors	Study Objective	Study Design	Findings
Kiley et al., 1993	Assessment of compliance with dietary and medication regimens post kidney transplant	Observational data on a series of 105 patients (27 white, 54 black, 21 Hispanic, 3 Asian) who received a kidney transplant at an urban university hospital during a 2-year period; follow-up was 18 to 55 months; mean 34.6 months	Black patients were underrepresented among patients compliant to both diet and medication; Hispanic patients were compliant to both diet and medication or to neither.
Wylie-Rosett et al., 1993	Efficacy of low sodium/high potassium diet or of weight reduction alone or in combination with medications for hypertension management	Ethnic comparison at 6 months of an intensive randomized trial of dietary intervention with 582 men and women (324 white and 158 black); participants were mildly hypertensive (DBP 90 to 100 mmHg), overweight (110 to 160% of MLIC standard weight), and off antihypertenisve medications for at least 2 weeks	Significantly fewer black participants achieved deitary goals for sodium and potassium.

Kumanyika et al., 1993	Efficacy of sodium reduction in preventing high blood pressure	Multicenter randomized controlled trial of sodium reduction in 30- to 54-year-old men and women with DBP between 80 and 89 mmHg at baseline	Black participants were significantly less likely than white participants to achieve the sodium reduction goal.
Wing and Anglin, 1996	Randomized comparison of weight loss in two different yearlong treatment programs	Treatments were a behavioral program with a low calorie diet throughout or which included two 12-week periods of a very low-calorie diet over 1 year	Blacks lost less weight, reported smaller initial changes in calorie intake, and had lower attendance than whites.
Van Horn et al., 1997	Cardiovascular disease risk reduction in high-risk men	Analyses of direct and indirect adherence measures, including modeling of baseline factors as adherence predictors	Blacks had poorer dietary adherence and smaller decreases in serum cholesterol than whites, while the reverse was true for Asians.

Note: TOHP = Trials of hypertension prevention; MLIC = Metropolitan Life Insurance Company

Source: Kumanyika, S.K., Minority populations, in *Compliance in Healthcare and Research*, Burke, L.E. and Ockene, I.S., Eds., Armonk, NY: Futura Publishing, 2001, Chap. 12.

Table 9.3   Examples of Studies Designed for Effectiveness with Minority Populations

Author	Program Focus and Population	Description	Evaluation
Cousins et al., 1992	Weight reduction in Mexican American women (n = 169 overweight women, ages 18 to 45) who were married and had at least one preschool aged child.	A behavior change manual, "Guidando el Corazon" and cookbook were developed to facilitate an eating plan low in total and saturated fat and weight reduction. The cookbook was based on typical Mexican American foods in Texas. Both Spanish and English versions of the materials were available. Individual treatment consisted of 24 weekly and then 6 monthly classes led by bilingual dietitians. Family treatment used the same approach but included information for partners, encouragement of spouses to attend, and separate classes for preschool children.	Participants were stratified on weight and randomly assigned to receive the manual only (control) or to treatment on an individual vs. family basis. A linear trend toward weight loss in all groups was observed, with the significant improvements in both the family and individual treatment groups (greater in the family group, but not significantly so) compared to the control group.

| Turner et al., 1995 | Church-based CVD health promotion in a rural county in North Florida; annual participation at church-based health promotion activities was 294 in year 1 and 343 (89% of the year 1 participanats plus 81 new participants); 68% women. | A Health Advisory Council of local church leaders was formed and guided by staff in the development of a program; the HAC reviewed background information on successful health programs, conducted a needs assessment from vital statistics data and a survey of local health problems, and developed a model program. Staff conducted heath promotion workshops to facilitate program development by church leaders. Prgorams involved medial publicity, a fashion show, cooking demonstrations, an exercise videctape to church music (Gospelsize), and nutrition and mental health awareness activities. The Council facilitated these activities, including development or identification of readily accessible resource materials. | High participant rates indicated achievement of the goal of increasing community; weekly exercise classes were among the most popular activities; systolic and diastolic blood pressure decreased in year 2 vs. year 1; improvements in dietary practices and physical activity were observed, although not all behavioral changes were statistically significant. |

Continued.

Table 9.3 Examples of Studies Designed for Effectiveness with Minority Populations (*Continued*)

Author	Program Focus and Population	Description	Evaluation
Flores 1995	Aerobic exercise program for low-income African American and Hispanic adolescents (n = 81; 54% female); 43% were Hispanic, 44% were African American, and 13% other ethnicity; 41% spoke Spanish at home; mean age was 12.6 years	Dance for Health was a dance-oriented physical activity curriculum developed to replace regular school physical education classes (mostly playground activities) for 7th grade students; attendance was mandatory, as for the regular class; students from each ethnic group were invited to recommend popular music; in addition, Dance for Health students attended health eduation classes (adapted from a cardiovascular disease education curriculum) twice a week and aerobics three times a week.	Classes were randomized to Dance for Health or regular physical education over 12 weeks. Dance for Health was associated with lower BMI, heart rate, improved fitness, and these changes were stastically significant in the girls. Girls in Dance for Health also had improved attitudes toward physical activity, but boys' attitudes worsened.

| Narayan et al., 1996 | Lifestyle intervention for NIDDM prevention in Pima Indians in Arizona (n = 95) overweight, non-diabetic men and women ages 25 to 54 years | Pima Pride emphasized self-directed learning and included monthly small group discussions of Pima culture, history, and current lifestyles. Written materials included a newsletter and basic nutrition and exercise information; Pima Action was a more conventional and more structured program with active encouragement to change diet and activity patterns through behaviorally oriented weekly group meetings and home visits as warranted. | Individuals were randomized to one of the two programs and re-examined at 6 and 12 months. Feedback on weight, glucose and serum cholesterol was provided at follow-up visits. An additional observational group of individuals who had refused randomization was also followed; both interventions were associated with increases in physical activity, and starch intake decreased in those in Pride. Several clinical measures, including weight, worsened in Action compared to Prides; clinical indicators also worsened in the observational group; program satisfaction was greater for Pride. |

Continued.

Table 9.3 Examples of Studies Designed for Effectiveness with Minority Populations (Continued)

Author	Program Focus and Population	Description	Evaluation
Kumanyika et al., 1999	Cardiovascular nutrition education for African Americans with diverse literacy skills (n = 244 women and 86 men; mean age 55 years); all participants had high blood pressure or high cholesterol	The CARDES prgram nutrition counseling materials were developed for use in outpatient settings; core items were a boxed deck of 100 food picture cards depicting typical servings of commonly eaten foods and included African American ethnic foods and an accompanying booklet with replicas of the cards and additional nutrition guidance. For a non-quantitative approach, cards were coded with symbols to indicate low, medium, or high content of fat, cholesterol, and sodium. A video and 12-program audioseries about an African American extended family were also developed to motivate behavior change and provide specific dietary change instructions in a vignette format.	Individuals were randomized to receive the full CARDES package or only the food cards and booklet. All participants received brief counseling by a nutritionist and feedback on their blood pressure and serum cholesterol; full instruction participants attended one class each month for the first four months. Follow-up at 12 months was complete for 77%. Both formats were associated with significant improvements in lipid profiles in women; men had better lipid results with full instruction; blood pressure improved for those with elevated blood pressure at baseline; outcomes did not differ by literacy level but were linked to the initial frequency of using the CARDES materials.

Source: Kumanyika, S.K., Minority populations, in *Compliance in Healthcare and Reserach*, Burke, L.E. and Ockene, I.S., Eds., Armonk, NY: Futura Publishing, 2001, Chap. 12.

nonethnic approach for all groups, regardless of ethnicity. Results from these data show differences in ethnicity relative to initial enrollment and provide dropout rates in follow-up stages of the study.

Table 9.3 is important because it illustrates ways to evaluate study interventions that are tailored to ethnicity within the context of lifestyle change. The cultural values, norms, and preferences are used to individualize the intervention.

Examples of ethnicity differences are seen in African American families where extended families are more interconnected with less of a distinct family unit than the usual American family. Also, African American families are often characterized as having a higher proportion of females as heads of the households [7]. For this type of female-dominated family structure where family members are interconnected, interventions that focus on the individual might be less effective. Kumanyika and Morssink note results from a study by Walden et al. where the research focused on African American girls and dietary adherence [8, 9]. Working with mother and daughter together resulted in a more highly positive intervention with the two working together in a supportive atmosphere. This is in contrast to work by Brownell where he studied Caucasian girls in which the mother and daughter together condition was inhibiting [10].

We used separate counseling in the mother and adolescent in the Diet Intervention Study in Children, Study of Nutrition in Teens, and the TREK study (described in Chapter 4). In each of these middle-class Caucasian populations, we worked with parents and teens in a separate fashion, yielding excellent dietary adherence rates. The separate session approach, where teens were more autonomous, was a structure that complemented the existing family dynamics.

In the WHI, an analysis of dietary adherence in an elderly group of women showed that factors associated with poorer dietary adherence included being African American or Hispanic as compared to Caucasian. Also associated with poorer adherence were the following characteristics: being older, having low income, and being obese [11].

9.2   IDENTIFYING YOUR PATIENT'S DESIRES

We often assume patient preferences without questioning their true desires. For example, in the WHI we assumed that study participants would be excited to work in small groups to prepare dishes reduced in fat. After surveying the participants we found that their first choice would be to watch the nutrition counselor demonstrate low-fat recipe preparation techniques. This one small desire on the part of the participants became a constant in each of the group sessions we designed and was a major reason for attendance by our study participants.

Table 9.4 Tailoring Adherence Stragies

Strategies	Methods of Tailoring
Modeling	Model preparation of quick, four-ingredient dessert parfait
Self-Monitoring	Include two simple forms of self-monitoring that allow for a check-off of items (i.e., number of servings of fruits and vegetables)
Self-Management	Negotiate an action plan, when the patient is ready for this stage, that involves managing the number of times a regular diet beverage was selected

9.3 IDENTIFYING YOUR PATIENT'S NEEDS

Patients' needs vary over time with changes in life events. To maintain lifestyle change, a thorough understanding of patients' needs is mandatory. Often it is necessary to streamline dietary adherence goals while patients struggle with devastating life events. As life events come into play and affect lifestyle behavior change, the ability of the nutrition counselor to be flexible is crucial to eventual high levels of dietary adherence. This kind of tailoring focuses on the realization that a small step backward in level of goal attainment might result in greater elevations in adherence at a later point in time when life events affecting nutrition lifestyle are more stable.

9.4 TAILORING STRATEGIES

Numerous strategies exist to facilitate excellent adherence to dietary regimens. The key to making a strategy a success in fostering adherence to diet is the level of tailoring that is used to ensure that a patient follows the strategy. Examples of strategies and methods of tailoring them appear in Table 9.4.

9.5 TAILORING MESSAGES

Often messages we give patients are generic and not individualized to the patient. For example, suggesting that eating out is a problem for everyone and providing strategies to improve selections is too generic when eating out might be the solution according to the nutrition counselor but not the solution according to the patient. Even if eating out is voiced as a problem by the patient, until the patient is ready to work on the problem, the action plan is a futile strategy designed to frustrate both the patient and nutrition counselor. Tailoring necessitates the acknowledgment by the patient that the action targeted is something achievable from his or her point of view.

Campbell has developed personalized newsletters that focus on an action plan where the patient identifies the nutrition lifestyle change area [12]. Campbell's work shows that tailoring a message in this way results in dietary behavior change.

9.6 USING TAILORING IN GROUP SETTINGS

Tailoring is also possible in group settings. Participants in a group negotiate an area of nutrition lifestyle change they would like to work on, and that becomes the focus. Often persons in the group who are successful in making change in that area become positive leaders for change for group members who are having difficulty. For example, the group decides to focus on portion sizes. One member of the group describes how she reduces portion sizes when she eats out: "I just ask for a take-home container after ordering my meal and then remove 1/3 of everything on my plate."

The importance of tailoring to patient needs is a paramount feature of nutrition counseling for lifestyle change. The factors discussed above focus on areas to observe and respond to, potentially resulting in the maximum success following nutrition counseling.

REFERENCES

1. Baughcum, A.E. et al., Maternal feeding practices and beliefs and their relationships to overweight in early childhood, *J. Dev. Behav. Pediatr.*, 22, 391, 2001.
2. Melgar-Quiñonez, H. and Kaiser, L., Relationship of feeding practices to overweight to low-income Mexican American preschool-age children, *J. Am. Diet. Assoc.*, 104, 110, 2004.
3. Robinson, T.N. et al., Is parental control over children's eating associated with childhood obesity? Results from a population-based sample of third graders, *Obes. Res.*, 9, 306, 2001.
4. Wardle, J. et al., Parental feeding style and the inter-generational transmission of obesity risk, *Obes. Res.*, 10, 453, 2002.
5. Airhihenbuwa, C.O., *Health and Culture*, Thousand Oaks, CA: Sage Publications, 1995.
6. Kumanyika, S.K., Minority populations, in *Compliance in Healthcare and Research*, Burke, L.E. and Ockene, I.S., Eds., Armonk, NY: Futura Publishing, 2001, Chap. 12.
7. Pollard, K.M. and O'Hare, W.P., America's racial and ethnic minorities, *Population Bulletin* 54.3, Washington DC: Population Reference Bureau, 1999.

8. Kumanyika, S.K. and Morssink, C.B., Cultural appropriateness of weight management programs, in *Overweight and Weight Management*, Dalton, S., Ed., Gaithersburg, MD: Aspen Publisher, 1997, 69–106.

9. Walden, T.A. et al., Obesity in black adolescent girls: a controlled clinical trial of treatment by diet, behavior modification and parental support, *Pediatrics*, 85, 345, 1990.

10. Brownell, K.D., Kelman, J.H., and Stunkard, A.J., Treatment of obese children with and without mothers: changes in weight and blood pressure, *Pediatrics*, 71, 515, 1983.

11. Women's Health Initiative Study Group, Dietary adherence in the women's Health Initiative Dietary Modification Trial, *J. Am. Diet. Assoc.*, 104, 654, 2004.

12. Campbell, M.K. et al., Improving dietary behavior: the effectiveness of tailored messages in primary care settings, *Am. J. Pub. Health*, 84, 783, 1994.

10

EXAMPLES OF DIETARY STRATEGIES BASED ON LONG-TERM RANDOMIZED CLINICAL TRIALS FOCUSED ON LIFESTYLE CHANGE

It becomes very obvious that nutrition lifestyle change is not an easy process for those patients requiring lifelong change. Just knowing what to eat based on current literature and research has little effect on actual patient eating habits. Changes in nutrition lifestyle to accommodate more healthful eating habits requires that the nutrition counselor understand patient priorities. Most patients have difficulty with change because they are influenced by the meaning food has to them and its effect on their value system. Our goal as nutrition counselors is to meld those individual meanings of food with the scientific knowledge we have of how food affects disease. In our present society the information overload includes so many controversial messages about food that the ability to change lifestyle is further complicated by confusion.

With current media providing the lay person with information that indicates the risks of not eating in a healthy fashion, it might seem obvious that nutrition lifestyle change is a positive. Additionally, one might assume that change would not be contested by patients as we work to modify their lifestyle relative to healthy eating habits. However, the opposite is true.

In a wonderfully written book on nutrition counseling, Katharine R. Curry and Amy Jaffe put thoughts to text describing why patients have difficulty in changing their nutrition lifestyle [1]. A few of the reasons why people have difficulty changing food habits is listed below:

1. Desire to equate food with love
2. Rebelliousness
3. A history of denying problems
4. Psychological illnesses
5. Depression and anxiety
6. Interpersonal relationships that might be affected negatively if nutrition lifestyle changes
7. Lack of immediate results reflecting positive outcomes
8. Overwhelming time and cost associated with extended treatment

Given these negatives relative to nutrition lifestyle change, what might the nutrition counselor do to modify a nutrition counseling plan to make it more efficient and effective? Below are four selected strategies that have been used in long-term clinical trials: (1) knowledge and skills, (2) feedback, (3) modeling, and (4) support and patient-centered counseling, which includes self-management and self-monitoring [2].

10.1 KNOWLEDGE AND SKILLS STRATEGIES

Nutrition interventions focus on nutrients in foods. It might be difficult for patients to determine what foods to select if they are not familiar with the nutrients in foods. This makes knowledge about the nutrient quantities in foods important. The ability of the counselor to provide this information requires the understanding of interests, needs, and adherence levels of individual participants. In the Modification of Renal Disease Study, participants were taught and practiced food record completion and self-monitoring techniques [2]. Participants also learned to discriminate foods by protein content, including learning skills in the use of a gram weight scale.

Likewise, in the Women's Health Initiative and the Women's Intervention Nutrition studies, women learned a great deal about the fat content of foods using a booklet that provided fat gram values for foods [3, 4]. The group sessions were designed to encourage reduced fat intake and increases in fruits and vegetables and grains. Each group session was tailored to the needs of the participants in the study. For example, often sessions described the nutritional benefits of certain types of fruits and vegetables. The types of fruits and vegetables focused on in dishes for sampling were those most available to women in the state or area where the women resided [3]. This data often indicated what types of foods were focused on as total fat was reduced. Different regions in the country may have included a different focus relative to food selections. With this knowledge, the dietitian could focus attention on those food groups that provided fat in that locale, with ideas for change specific to that participant population.

In the Diabetes and Control Complications Trial (DCCT), the focus was on achieving blood glucose levels that were in normal ranges. The protocol for this study focused on the goal of achieving a normal HbA1C. Any route to that goal was approved. This meant that within the 29 centers involved in the DCCT, several different plans were used for dietary instruction [5]. The plans included Healthy Food Choices, The Exchange System, Carbohydrate Counting, and Total Available Glucose. In this study, participants were fine-tuning insulin to the carbohydrate in foods they ate. The focus in the DCCT was on pre-meal or pre-prandial blood glucose. The use of both Healthy Food Choices and The Exchange System had the potential for making pre-meal insulin boluses less precise. For both Carbohydrate Counting and Total Available Glucose, the precision of insulin adjustment was increased. With carbohydrate counting, insulin dose was adjusted based on the ratio of regular insulin to grams of carbohydrate intake. For total available glucose, insulin dose was adjusted based on the ratio of regular insulin to total available glucose (carbohydrate + 58% protein + 10% fat) eaten. For each of these methods, knowledge and skills were necessary.

In the Diet Intervention Study in Children, both children and parents were given information on the saturated fat content of foods that children and adolescents love. Each family was given a saturated fat booklet that included brand name and fast food restaurant products. Fun sessions were designed with adults in one area and children and adolescents in another to present single concepts in tailored ways for children and adolescents, and adults [6, 7].

10.2 FEEDBACK

Feedback is very important within each stage. The act of presenting information about laboratory values and dietary intake over time allows the patient to analyze for himself or herself when problems occurred [8, 9]. It is a way of self assessing what lifestyle change might have fostered changes in dietary behavior. For the patient to assess what is happening apart from the counselor telling the story, a more tailored realization of problems occurs. There is less resentment on the part of the patient and a greater feeling of control when the feedback and its analysis are in the hands of the patient [2].

10.3 MODELING

Often our best planned counseling strategies fail to be used because the patient has not been shown how to use the strategy. This concept of modeling a behavior is extremely important in lifestyle change related to dietary behaviors. Bandura was one of the first to describe the concept of modeling. It is an important strategy used in the psychological model of social learning theory [10, 11]. As counselors we often focus on what we believe the patient should know. The truth is that our ideas of their level of understanding might be much higher than is actually true. Bandura describes modeling as a four-step process that includes: (1) observation, (2) remembering, (3) reproduction, and (4) feedback. Observation is illustrated when a nutrition counselor demonstrates the preparation of a recipe in a group setting. The goal with modeling recipe preparation allows patients to visualize preparation techniques. This visualizing assists in remembering what to do, and in combination with a written recipe, it is more likely to ensure use of the recipe at home. To further ensure comfort with recipe preparation, allowing patients to help while preparation occurs shows the ability to reproduce preparation at an individual level. This reproduction step also allows the nutritionist to provide positive constructive feedback to further ensure use of the recipe at home.

Examples of each life stage and a modeling of healthy eating behaviors are provided in Table 10.1.

Table 10.1 Modeling within Life Stages

Life Stages	Modeling
Stage 1: Childhood and Parental Feeding Habits	Parents model the importance of foods high in nutrients by eating fruits and vegetables with their children.
Stage 2: Children and Adolescents	Children and teens eat fruits and vegetables in school through a special program designed to provide fruits and vegetables.
Stage 3: Adults and the Elderly	Busy and stressed adults and elderly persons as part of group sessions learn from other participants describing how they focused on identifying feelings and dealing with them using appropriate coping strategies, not overeating or eating in an unhealthy manner.

10.4 SUPPORT AND PATIENT-CENTERED COUNSELING

Many of the interventions completed with changing nutrition lifestyle in long-term randomized clinical trials are focused on patient-centered approaches. These approaches include two important theories of change: social cognitive theory [12, 13] and stages of change theory [14–17]. Evidence from three randomized clinical trials shows that the patient-centered model is effective. These studies include: a dietary randomized controlled clinical trial (RCT) or Watch [18], an alcohol RCT or Project Health [19], and a smoking RCT conducted by Ockene and colleagues [20].

10.4.1 Self-Management

The patient who learns to self-manage becomes the expert in problem solving. This translates into a skill that allows constant checks and changes as the patient applies healthy behaviors in real-life situations. The goal is to facilitate the concept that the patient is the expert and does not have to constantly rely on someone else to direct his or her every move. This kind of new-found empowerment makes the patient feel in control, which is a very gratifying feeling. It eliminates the concern that something is wrong, and the patient has no power to modify the situation to improve nutrition lifestyle habits.

10.4.2 Self-Monitoring

Patients can learn how to self-monitor. In the Women's Health Initiative, participants in the study self-monitored at various levels [21]. The instruments used are described in Table 10.2. Although self-monitoring initially gives an overall picture of all eating habits throughout a day, it does not need to continue at this all-inclusive level throughout the counseling period. This crucial part of self-management does not have to be done at the most complicated level as lifestyle change progresses. This type of data is available for the patient to see how well adherence to a new eating pattern is progressing. Often if behaviors are very specific, as they should be, they are monitored in a focused fashion (i.e., number of servings of fruits and vegetables, number of grams of saturated fat, or number and types of snacks before bed). Self-monitoring is a key factor in self-management because it is a skill that allows patients to self-correct and make adjustments in lifestyle change.

Chapters 5, 6, and 7 review the process of stages of change and give very specific examples of ways to use this theoretical construct in modifying nutrition lifestyle behavior. When the patient is at a level of change that will allow goal setting, self-monitoring should be tied to specific goals.

Table 10.2 WHI Self-Monitoring Instruments

	Food Diary	Fat Scan	Mini Diary	Keeping Track of Goals	Quick Scan	Picture Tracker	Eating Pattern Changes
Description	Space is provided to write each food eaten; columns allow for tallying fat grams and servings of fruits, vegetables, and grains.	250 foods are listed by food group having greatest impact on fat intake; fat grams are listed with servings of fruits and vegetables.	This is a miniature version of the larger food diary.	There is a letter and pocket-size version to record fat grams and servings of fruit, vegetables, and grains.	This instrument included selected foods most commonly chosen from the fat scan; a computerized version was available.	Fruit, vegetables, and grain icons are included to circle based on number of servings consumed; room is available to list low- and high-fat foods but not to record fat grams.	Questionnaire is designed to assess low-fat eating habits and identify goals.
Number of days per booklet or sheet	7	3	18	6–18	3	1 day/page	Ad lib period of time

Sources: Mossavar-Rahmani et al., *J. Am. Diet. Assoc.*, 104, 76, 2004; Tinker et al., in *Nutrition in Women's Health*, Gaithersburg, MD: Aspen, 1966, 510–542.

A crucial part of goal setting is negotiating the nutrition lifestyle change with the patient. Although many counselors would like to impose their goals on patients, and often they might have very good instincts for the most productive direction a patient might follow, the counselor's goals are not the goals that will work in all cases for all patients. Goal setting for nutrition lifestyle change should be a partnership with the patient and nutrition counselor working together.

REFERENCES

1. Curry, K.R. and Jaffe, A., *Nutrition Counseling and Communication Skills,* Philadelphia, PA: W.B. Saunders Company, 1998, 6–7.
2. Gillis, B.P., Caggiula, A.W., Chiavacci, A.T., Coyne, T., Doroshenko, L., Milas, C., Nowalk, P., and Scherch, L.K., Nutrition intervention program of the Modification of Diet in Renal Disease Study: A self-management approach, *J. Am. Diet. Assoc.,* 95, 1288–1294, 1995.
3. Patterson, R.E., Kristal, A.R., Coates, R.J., Tylavsky, F.A., Ritenbaugh, C., Van Horn, L., Caggiula, A.W., and Snetselaar, L., Low-fat diet practices of older women: prevalence and implications for dietary assessment, *J. Am. Diet. Assoc.,* 96, 670, 1996.
4. Winters, B.L., Mitchell, D.C., Smiciklas-Wright, H., Grosvenor, M.B., Liu, W., and Blackburn, G.L., Dietary patterns in women treated for breast cancer who successfully reduce fat intake: The Women's Intervention Nutrition Study (WINS), *J. Am. Diet. Assoc.,* 104, 551, 2004.
5. The DCCT Research Group, Nutrition interventions for intensive therapy in the Diabetes Control and Complications Trial, *J. Am. Diet. Assoc.,* 93, 768, 1993.
6. Stevens, V.J., Obarzanek, E., Franklin, F.A., Steinmuller, P., Snetselaar, L., Lavigne, J., Batey, D., von Almen, T.K., Hartmuller, V., Reimers, T., Lasser, V.I., Craddick, S., and Gernhofer, N., Dietary Intervention Study in Children (DISC): intervention design and participation, *J. Nutr. Ed.,* 27, 133, 1995.
7. Van Horn, L., Stumbo, P., Moag-Stahlberg, A., Obarzanek, E., Hartmuller, V.W., Farris, R., Kimm, S.U.S., Frederick, M., and Snetselaar, L., The Dietary Intervention Study in Children (DISC): dietary assessment methods for 8- to 10-year-olds, *J. Am. Diet. Assoc.,* 93, 1396, 1993.
8. Berg-Smith, S.M., Stevens, V.J., Brown, K.M., Van Horn, L., Gernhofer, N., Peters, E., Greenberg, R., Snetselaar, L., Ahrens, L., and Smith, K., for the Dietary Intervention Study in Children (DISC) Research Group, A brief motivational intervention to improve dietary adherence in adolescents, *Health Ed. Res.,* 14, 399, 1999.
9. Bowen, D., Ehret, C., Pedersen, M., Snetselaar, L., Johnson, M., Tinker, L., Hollinger, D., Lichty, I., Bland, K., Sivertsen, D., Ocken, D., Staats, L., and Williams Beedoe, J., Results of an adjunct dietary intervention program in the Women's Health Initiative, *J. Am. Diet. Assoc.,* 102, 1631, 2002.
10. Bandura, A., *Social Learning Theory,* Englewood Cliffs, NJ: Prentice-Hall, 1977.
11. Bandura, A., *Self-efficacy: The Exercise of Control,* New York: WH Freeman and Company, 1997.
12. Bandura, A., Self-efficacy: toward a unifying theory of behavioral change, *Psychol. Rev.,* 84, 191, 1977.

13. Bandura, A., Self-efficacy mechanism in physiological activation and health-promoting behavior, in *Neurobiology of Learning, Emotion and Affect*, Madden, J., Ed., New York: Raven Press, 1991, 229–270.
14. Prochaska, J. and DiClemente, C., Stages and processes of self-change of smoking: toward an integrative model of change, *J. Consult. Clin. Psych.*, 51, 390–395, 1983.
15. Horn, D., A model for the study of personal choice health behavior, *J. Health Educ.*, 19, 89–98, 1976.
16. Lichtenstein, E. and Brown, R., Smoking cessation methods: review and recommendations, in *Addictive Behaviors: Treatment of Alcoholism, Drug Abuse, Smoking and Obesity*, Miller, W., Ed., New York: Pergamon Press, 1980.
17. Ockene, J.K., Strategies to increase adherence to treatment, in *Compliance in Healthcare and Research*, Burke, L.E. and Ockene, I.S., Eds., Armonk, NY: Futura Publishing Company, 2001, Chap. 2.
18. Ockene, J.K., Herbert, H., and Ockeene, J. et al., Effect of physician-delivered nutrition counseling training and a structured office-support program on saturated fat intake, weight, and serum lipid measurements in a hyperlipidemic population: Worcester Area Trial for Counseling in Hyperlipidemia (WATCH), *Arch. Intern. Med.*, 159, 725, 1999.
19. Ockene, J.K., Wheeler, E., and Adams, A. et. al., Provider training for patient-centered alcohol counseling in a primary care setting, *Arch. Intern. Med.*, 157, 2334, 1997.
20. Ockene, J.K., Kristeller, J., and Pbert, L. et al., The PDSIP: can short-term interventions produce long-term effects for a general outpatient population, *Health Psychol.*, 14, 278, 1994.
21. Mossavar-Rahmani, Y., Henry, H., Rodabough, R., Bragg, C., Brewer, A., Freed, T., Kinzel, L., Pedersen, M., and Soule, O., Additional self-monitoring tools in the dietary modification component of the Women's Health Initiative, *J. Am. Diet. Assoc.*, 104, 76, 2004.
22. Tinker, L.F., Burrows, E.R., Henry, H., Patterson, R., Rupp, J., and Van Horn, L., The Women's Health Initiative: overview of the nutrition components, in *Nutrition in Women's Health*, Krummel, D. and Kris-Etherton, P., Eds., Gaithersburg, MD: Aspen, 1996, 510–542.

11

REDUCING STRESS TO MAINTAIN DIETARY CHANGE

11.1 DEFINITION OF STRESS

Stress is a major portion of daily life. It includes those pressures that come naturally as our patients deal with life's changes and events, such as children leaving home, new schools, illnesses, getting married, changing jobs. Stress is not always bad for our patients. Stress can facilitate major accomplishments. As we work with patients it is important to realize that pressure and tension can trigger both good and bad stress.

11.2 IDENTIFYING STRESS

A patient's response to stress can be physiological, resulting in muscle strain and tension, headaches, and indigestion. Additionally it can result in altered responses to situations that involve our thoughts and emotional reactions. Persons under stress are more likely to react with irritability and anger. Often some of the first indicators of stress are depression and unrealistic concern about the possibility of distressful events. A person's reaction to stress can result in over- and undereating or drinking.

For a nutrition counselor, these very different responses to stress are important because the concept of tailoring strategies to each individual patient becomes important. Situations that are stressful for some might be adventurous and pleasant for others. Often the critical factor in dealing with stressful circumstances is the lack of control or ability to cope with an event that might lead to dangerous, painful, or difficult outcomes.

The inability to control what might seem like an inevitable situation can affect eating habits in very different ways. For some patients it will result in uncontrolled eating binges and for others total abstinence from eating. Additionally, required changes in dietary habits can lead to stressful family responses if the change is negative for them. This dietary change becomes the reason for stress for many patients.

Reactions to stress can be behavioral, physical, and emotional as mentioned previously. Different reactions are listed below:

Behavioral:

Sleeplessness
Lack of attentiveness resulting in proneness toward accidents
Loss of appetite
Increase in eating or drinking without regard for hunger signals

Physical:

Headaches
Indigestion or diarrhea
Grinding teeth
Breathlessness
Dizziness
Trembling

Emotional:

Lack of concentration
Anger
Irritability
Negative affect
Depression
Unwarranted worry

Probes to use in questioning patients are focused on what outcomes occur when stress is high and how patients have dealt with stress in the past. Many patients deal with stress in inappropriate ways. This is a result of modeling through life events by peers and parents earlier in life. The nutrition counselor addresses this problem by asking a variety of questions:

What do you usually do in a stressful situation? This question is very open and allows the patient to respond with detail around those situations that are particularly memorable.

How has changing your nutrition lifestyle changed stress for you? Do you devote extra time to purchasing and preparing food? Do you feel deprived? Do you think about food more often and is eating less spontaneous? Does a family's food preference make it difficult to eat healthy

Table 11.1 Modifying Favorite Foods to Add Zest

Vinegar and Mustard

Try flavored vinegars such as raspberry, balsamic, or herbed.
Use seasoned rice vinegar as a dressing.
Dijon mustard and other hot mustards add flavor to marinades and sauces.

Peppers

Use milder peppers (bell peppers, New Mexican, and ancho).
Try hot peppers (jalapeno, Serrano, habanero).

Herbs and Spices

Experiment with basil, oregano, thyme, and bay leaves.
Add interest with curry powder, garlic, or ginger.
Add zest with pepper, cayenne, cilantro, or red pepper flakes.

Modified from Session 17, Ver. 2: 06/30/95, Women's Health Initiative.

foods? Are social events difficult due to the changes in your dietary pattern? Recognizing stress and its affect on lifestyle can help the nutrition counselor point to new ways of coping.

Asking the following question can elicit ideas that are tailored to individual needs: "What do you do to reduce stress when it affects your eating habits?" Past strategies will provide the nutrition counselor with clues to help in providing examples of ways to cope.

11.3 STRATEGIES TO REDUCE STRESS

As a nutrition counselor the objectives behind reducing stress may include many types of situations that might result in inappropriate eating habits. First, training patients to deal with anticipated stress and then tolerate it when it happens can help in alleviating impulse eating that is often not appropriately healthy. For example, if a reunion is approaching where many dishes will be too high in calories, coaching the patient on how to prepare a favorite dish in a healthy manner so that at least one offering at the reunion is appropriate might be a suggestion. Table 11.1 provides examples of how to modify favorite foods.

A second goal that is often used to reduce stress around food is that of providing techniques to help patients recover from distressing episodes more rapidly and completely by minimizing their aftereffects. For the nutrition counselor this means that offering ideas related to streamlining tasks associated with adhering to the diet are very important. Providing quick, easy-to-prepare meals might help when dealing with the aftermath

Table 11.2   Quick Meals

Plan ahead by stocking your pantry and freezer with necessary ingredients for healthy, quick meals.

Ideas:
- Spaghetti with bottled or canned tomato sauce
- Canned chili
- Packaged macaroni and cheese made with skim milk and without margarine or half the margarine
- Pork n' beans with brown bread
- Microwaved potato topped with cottage cheese and vegetables
- Frozen ravioli with bottled or canned tomato sauce
- Refrigerated mashed potatoes with broccoli and salsa
- Fresh finger food fruits and vegetables
- Stir fried chicken with frozen vegetables
- Soup and sandwich
- Microwaved fish with salsa

Modified from Session 15, Ver. 2: 06/30/95, Women's Health Initiative.

of stress that leaves the patient feeling fatigued and uninterested in meal preparation. Table 11.2 provides ideas for quick meals as an example of what might be used in dietary intervention sessions.

A third objective in dealing with stress involves the concept of dealing with daily tensions that can alter eating habits. Offering healthy meals when eating on the run can be of value in this situation. Providing ideas on healthy fast foods, such as McDonald's apples and yogurt or parfait with fruit and salads might spark the desire to use fast food establishments to their advantage.

Time management and planning ahead are often considered essential when dealing with stressful eating situations. These two strategies help with organizing and prioritizing daily eating style.

Changes in goal setting are also important. Often patients will set unrealistic goals and try to be perfect in their eating habits. This can lead to a lack of success in meeting the goals and result in a more stressful situation.

11.4   TWO APPROACHES AND ORIENTATIONS

There are two major approaches when dealing with stress. The first is to change the environment by altering the stressor or reducing exposure to it. The ideas discussed previously are responses to the environment. The second is to change the patient's response to the stress. The first approach is problem-focused and the second approach is emotion-focused. These two approaches are complementary rather than mutually exclusive. In nutrition counseling both are important. However, new preliminary research described in Chapter 13 indicates that the emotion-focused approach might be more effective in maintaining weight loss. Identifying life as stressful can mask feelings that lead to overeating. Feelings do not need to be eliminated because identifying feelings can be helpful. The changes need to occur in the way a patient copes with feelings. Chapter 13 describes new untested theories related to feelings. In her book *The Solution*, Mellin describes stress as a smokescreen and states that identifying the feeling that accompanies stress and a coping strategy should be the focus [1].

Building on the objectives discussed above with the concept of problem- and emotion-focused stress management, strategies to deal with stress range from being assertive in expressing eating desires to dealing in an appropriate way with emotion-driven-eating cravings. The words "no thank you" can assist the patient in asserting will when trying to avoid certain foods.

Asking the patient what methods he or she currently uses to cope with stress can result in more useful collaborative goal setting. Knowing what coping strategies have worked in the past is a good predictor of what will work in the future.

In summary, keeping points related to stress simple is important. Below are just a few ideas that cover both the environmental and emotional orientation of stress management:

Use positive self-talk.
Plan ahead.
Use time-management skills.
Find a support system.
Set feasible goals.
Be assertive.

The discussions that follow are derived from actual experiences in the Women's Health Initiative Study [2].

11.4.1 Positive Self-Talk

Helping patients see the positive, even in slips from healthy eating, can eliminate the "all or nothing" attitude about healthy eating. The idea that perfection is the only way to success is identified as leading to erroneous expectations and eventual regression to past eating habits. Providing ideas to stop negative monologues, and replacing them with positive thoughts, can be very encouraging and provide ideas for dealing with negative situations in the future.

Table 11.3 provides some concepts that help in understanding positive self-talk and may allow the patient to see how to revise those internal emotion-driven thoughts in a positive direction. By identifying the coping strategies used as stressful situations occur, it is possible to turn those ideas that surface in emotional context to the positive. Often in the context of general stress it is easy to focus on the negative. Coping in a new way by using more positive self-talk can increase motivation to continue to strive for more healthful eating behaviors.

11.4.2 Planning Ahead

The concept of planning ahead is useful in preventing setbacks in healthful eating but also in providing ideas for future strategies to deal with problem situations. Planning ahead allows the patient to be in control as a stressful situation occurs. Bringing a favorite healthy dish to a reunion so that it might be the one dish chosen in the largest serving amount, is a strategy to help avoid making a reunion an eating disaster.

One of the participants in the Women's Health Initiative stated that she found a friend to talk with and sat as far away from the food as possible. This meant that she could thoroughly enjoy the event without eating more than she intended.

Other suggestions by participants have been to suggest to a friend that they take a walk around the area in which the reunion is occurring. This adds exercise, fun conversation, and a move from an event that can be totally food-focused.

11.4.3 Time-Management Skills

Time saving techniques include the important element of organization. Planning meals ahead can afford one time to focus on what types of foods would be appropriate. Keeping an ongoing shopping list provides a level of organization that mandates more healthy eating habits. Time-saving ingredients (pre-cut vegetable or boned skinless chicken) make the process of recipe preparation shorter. Healthy convenience foods (frozen, canned, or instant) allow for time-saving food preparation. Many patients have emphasized the importance of maintaining a quick and easy recipe file. Often pre-preparation for a meal is the first step in the time management process. Preparing part of the meal ahead of time makes actual meal preparation easier and less time-consuming. Making a double batch and freezing it for a later meal cuts down on preparation time. Often, one meal can be devised to be used for leftovers in another meal. Methods that shorten cooking time contribute to time management. These methods

Table 11.3 Concepts Related to Self-Talk

Self-Talk Categories	Patient-Oriented Description	Potential Responses	
		Negative Self-Talk	Positive Self-Talk
Overgeneralization	If it is true in this case, it applies to any case that is even slightly similar.	"I ate too many potato chips at the last party I attended, and I'll probably do the same here."	"This situation is different and I have learned new skills that I can use this time."
Self-Abstraction	The only events that matter are failures.	"Well I blew it when I ate that piece of cheesecake. This just isn't working for me. I might as well quit."	"Normally, I don't eat cheesecake. I only had one piece. I will be sure to eat more fruit as a snack and always have it available at home."
Excessive Responsibility	Slip = failure. I am responsible for all bad things.	"I am a failure. I knew I should have avoided the cookies."	"This is a single mistake, not a failure. I can use it to learn how to handle future high-stress situations."
Self-Reference	I am the center of everyone's attention, especially when I fail.	"If I didn't eat that last doughnut at work, my coworkers wouldn't think I'm such a failure."	"My coworkers are supportive, I'll ask them to help me the next time I am tempted to eat the last doughnut."
Catastrophizing	Always think the worst; it is likely to happen.	"I ate a piece of coconut cream pie, now my kids will never let me hear the end of it."	"I can explain to my kids that no foods are forbidden. I do not need to eat pie every day, and I stopped at one piece."
Dichotomous Thinking	Everything is one extreme or another.	"If I have one cookie, everything is lost."	"One more cookie will not break my healthy eating plan."
Willpower Breakdown	Willpower is absolute; once it has failed, loss of control is inevitable.	"I just have no more willpower."	"There are a lot of things I can do to control the amount and types of foods I eat."

Modified from WHI Manuals: Volume 4 — Dietary Modification Intervention.

might include stir-frying, poaching, and broiling. Using a convection oven, microwave, electric skillet, or pressure cooker can reduce cooking time.

11.4.4 Support Systems

Finding support in groups similar to those used in large-scale studies like the Women's Health Initiative can be beneficial to dietary adherence. Suggestions from those in like situations who attend group sessions show that adherence over time is possible in a population of women following a low-fat diet with increased fruits and vegetables and grains [2]. Group support can contribute to maintenance of dietary behaviors over long periods of time. In the article referenced above, excellent dietary adherence in postmenopausal women is reported for years 1 and 5.

11.4.5 Feasible Goals

Often goals that are unattainable will lead to stress and a lack of confidence in maintaining healthy eating behaviors. A major focus in setting goals should be the end result relative to outcomes. If the goals are not feasible, the motivation to continue striving for attainment is lessened. This in itself can be a stressor that leads to unhealthy eating habits.

11.4.6 Assertiveness

Learning to say "no thank you" is a most important skill when emotions are key to success. Feeling good about turning down a food that is not a favorite just to please a relative or friend is okay. It is important to let a patient know that it is okay to elicit the respect of those around him or her as decisions are made about eating.

The strategies related to reducing stress are numerous. Many have a basis in their positive effect on diet adherence in long-term randomized dietary-related trials.

REFERENCES

1. Mellin, L., *The Solution*, New York: Harper Collins, 1997, 158.
2. Women's Health Initiative Study Group, Dietary adherence in the Women's Health Initiative Dietary Modification Trial, *J. Am. Diet. Assoc.*, 104, 654, 2004.

12

ORGANIZING DATA ON DIETARY CHANGE

12.1   SETTING THE STAGE FOR ORGANIZATION

The organization of dietary data based on adherence to change in nutrition lifestyle can be of benefit in terms of designing nutrition intervention programs.

Because of the streamlining of the Prochaska/DiClemente model to include three stages of change — sure, unsure, and not ready to change — an automatic categorization of nutrition lifestyle change is available. This is one way of tailoring a nutrition intervention to a particular stage of readiness. Chapters 5, 6, and 7 provide specific ways of counseling for each stage of change in each lifecycle stage.

This method was not used in the Women's Health Initiative to classify adherence because other factors were also important as we worked to improve adherence. Table 12.1 describes the four levels of adherence to Women's Health Initiative goals, with 1 being best and 4 being worst. This system of numbering did not mean that for those doing well at level 1 no attention was given because that would lead to an increase in the level of categorization with reduced adherence to dietary lifestyle change. Likewise, too much emphasis on a person in level 4 might lead to no change and would be wasted effort. Levels 2 and 3 are the levels with most promise for improvement and movement to level 1.

Several factors were important to ultimate nutrition lifestyle change: attendance at sessions, self-monitoring, and compliance with the diet regimen including fat gram, fruit and vegetable servings, and grain servings. By classifying adherence data we have a way of identifying problems with all of the patients we are counseling. For groups, this will provide

Table 12.1 Four Levels of Dietary Adherence in Women's Health Initiative Participants

Triage staff efforts beginning with participants in Level 1 and ending with participants in Level 4. Focus time and effort on improving adherence to the fat gram goal and self-monitoring through Additional Assistance activities with participants in Levels 2 and 3.

Adherence Level	Staff Time and Effort	Participant Effort	Adherence Activities
1	★★	Completes sessions and meets fat gram goal	Reaffirm and encourage meeting fat gram goal
			Reward self-monitoring and session attendance by giving positive feedback.
2	★★★★	Completes sessions and self-monitors but does **not meet fat gram goal**	Conduct Additional Assistance using participant-centered counseling.
			Assess:
			■ Have participant identify problem(s) **interfering with reaching fat gram goal.**
			■ Discuss participant's readiness and confidence to change.
			Negotiate and Motivate:
			■ If ready to change, then negotiate a plan for change — have the participant identify the steps.
			■ If not ready to change, help the participant move closer to change — help the participant develop dissonance and explore ambivalence about change.
			Arrange:
			■ Work with the participant to arrange future contact.

---

3 · ★★★ · Completes sessions, but **does not self-monitor** · Conduct additional assistance using participant-centered counseling.

Assess:

- Have participant identify problem(s) **interfering with self monitoring.**
- Discuss participant's readiness and confidence to change.

Negotiate and Motivate:

- If ready to change, then negotiate a plan for change — have the participant identify the steps.
- If not ready to change, help the participant move closer to change — help the participant develop dissonance and explore ambivalence about change.

Arrange:

- Work with the participant to arrange contact.

Negotiate interrupted DM intervention participation.

4 · ★ · Completes 1 session

★ = no additional effort; ★★★ = extensive additional effort

a system of identifying similar problems. For individuals, it targets groups of problems that may affect subsets of those we are counseling.

Patient-centered counseling where the patient is involved in discussions around what might work to remediate nutrition lifestyle change problems is a key to achieving change. For example, in group counseling, those patients who are not attending sessions routinely might all be given an assessment of why attendance has tapered off. Additionally, patients might be asked what strategies they wish to use to increase attendance.

For those who need assistance with self-monitoring, new streamlined strategies might be used. Some of the most creative and useful self-monitoring tools have been designed by participants. One creative approach was designed around beads on a bracelet, where each time a gram of fat was eaten beads were moved to a different location on the bracelet. By the end of the day all of the beads should have been relocated, thus showing goal attainment. This creative approach to self-monitoring was something only a person who had dealt with real-life situations involving nutrition lifestyle change could have devised. The counselor who tries to have all of the answers often misses the creative talents of the individual she or he is trying to help.

12.2   PRESENTING DIETARY ADHERENCE DATA TO PATIENTS

An important element of motivational interviewing involves showing the patient his or her dietary adherence data and asking what has happened over time to create rises and falls in adherence. Figure 12.1 is an example of one patient's hypothetical dietary adherence over a period of 2 years. She kept records of her dietary fat intake 3 days a month. The records show changes in her lifestyle over 2 years that have affected her dietary habits.

12.3   INVOLVING THE PATIENT IN LIFESTYLE CHANGE DATA REVIEW

The goal is for the patient to assess the graph (Figure 12.1) and describe what happened as dietary adherence changed. Both positive and negative factors will result from an analysis of this data. Asking the patient to describe barriers to and resources for success is empowering and much more patient-centered than a process where the counselor analyzes data for the patient.

Below is a script of what might transpire as the patient reviews her data provided in Figure 12.1.

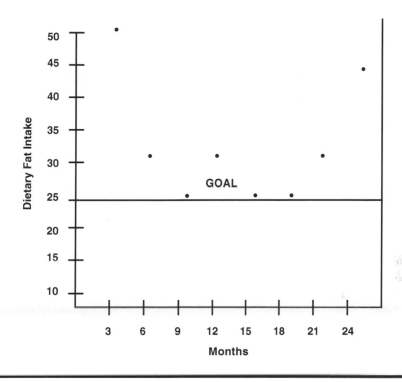

Figure 12.1   Dietary fat intake. Average of three days of dietary records for each of three months.

Nutrition Counselor: As you look at this graph what do you see in regard to your ability to meet your goal of 25 grams of fat per day?

Patient: I see that I have followed the diet as many times as I have not. I also know that there are times in my life when it has been more difficult to follow the diet; for example, at the 6-month point, which was when my husband was diagnosed with a heart condition. I had a difficult time then. My lifestyle changed and became very hectic. Then my husband had surgery and did well at 9 months, and I just wanted to be more spontaneous with my diet at 12 months.

Nutrition Counselor: What specific things made adherence more difficult for you when your fat intake went up?

Patient: Stress is a huge reason that I stop adhering. I just do not know how to deal with it and still follow my low-fat eating pattern.

Nutrition Counselor: You did much better at 12 months than at 3 months even though there was a rise in your fat intake. Why was that different?

Patient: I learned how to deal with stress by using relaxation therapy, and I learned how to deal with slips from the previous time when my fat intake skyrocketed. My reason for eating more fat was different at 12 months. I just decided that I wanted to be more spontaneous. Stress was less of a problem, and I felt more in control.

Nutrition Counselor: What specifically did you do to stay in control? How might you use this strategy to return to your goal now?

Patient: My husband is good at reminding me. He is a great support of my dietary changes. I also try to relax more about food and not feel panicked about always eating perfectly. I tend to do better if I stay calm. That would help me regain control now.

This dialogue shows how important it is to use patient-centered counseling and how important allowing the patient to express ideas is in the problem-solving process. Allowing the patient to use data to make changes is one way of maximizing our resources for dietary change.

13

POTENTIAL NEW THEORIES PLAYING A ROLE IN NUTRITION LIFESTYLE CHANGE

13.1 AFFECTIVE AND COGNITIVE FACTORS INFLUENCE WEIGHT CONTROL BEHAVIORS

New theories are becoming a focus as researchers work to find more successful ways of dealing with the obesity epidemic. We often look to the past to find research that shows potential for theories that might be applied to current treatment regimens. Studies have shown that increased eating in response to negative affect is common in persons with high levels of restraint [1–3]. Also, evidence is available to show that overweight persons consume more than normal or underweight persons during negative emotional periods in their lives [4, 5]. Schlundt, a psychologist who has worked with persons who have binge and disordered eating episodes, in surveying overweight persons has found that they rate their ability to cope with eating temptations during negative emotional states as less competent than normal weight persons [6]. The Eating Inventory provides an indicator of "disinhibition" and is a commonly used descriptive measure to analyze eating in response to social cues, cognitions, and emotions [7, 8]. Thus, eating in response to negative affect (feeling sad, deprived, stressed, less in control, anxious, angry, etc.) has been observed in persons who are classified as restrained eaters. Self-reported emotional eating is more often described in overweight vs. normal weight persons. Weight regain can be predicted by disinhibition of eating in response to emotion and cognitions.

13.2 NEGATIVE AFFECTIVE STATES AND DYSFUNCTIONAL COGNITIONS RELATED TO RELAPSE

Researchers show that half of the self-reported relapse following behavioral weight control treatments occurred when negative affect preceded the relapse [9, 10, 11]. While much of behavioral treatment is focused on environmental factors that affect lifestyle change, Grilo and colleagues have studied situations where negative affect is the primary precursor to an unhealthy food choice. They found that subjects in their study who described negative feelings prior to selecting unhealthy foods were more likely to relapse than to use coping skills to avoid the temptation [9].

Carels and colleagues used a methodology called ecological momentary assessment (EMA) to examine temptations and lapses in dieters who were attempting to reduce weight on their own [12]. Those researchers showed that there was a positive association between negative affect and temptations followed by lapses in healthy eating habits. EMA was also used in a study involving women who had just finished a behavioral weight loss program. This study showed that lapses were associated with self-reported negative feelings [13].

Byrne and his colleagues have shown that certain characteristics are associated with persons who regain weight [14]. Regainers often display a dichotomous thinking style, for example, "If I eat just one bite of this cheesecake, I have gone off my diet, and there is no hope for me." Also Byrne and his coresearchers observed that regainers respond to adverse life events by eating and use eating to distract themselves from negative feelings. In a prospective follow-up to this observational study, Byrne and coworkers found that in women who had achieved a 10% weight loss for 1 year in a community program, the strongest predictor of regain was a dichotomous thinking style [15].

Often in working with nutrition-related lifestyle change, depression is associated with weight gain and obesity. Obese persons report higher levels of depression than nonobese [16, 17]. It is interesting that in one study gender differences existed with a negative association between obesity in males and depression with positive associations between obesity in females and depression [18].

Often gender is important with two studies completed in women showing that increased BMI is associated with both suicidal tendencies and depression [19, 20]. Three prospective studies looking at risk factors for obesity show that obesity is a risk factor for depression [21] and that depression is a risk factor for weight gain [22, 23]. Again, Korkeila and colleagues showed gender differences [24]. Low life satisfaction was a predictor of weight gain in women with stress predicting weight gain in men.

Today with the focus on maintaining weight loss, the importance of affective and cognitive processes on weight control behaviors is acknowledged clinically, with some new research in this area beginning. Fairburn and colleagues have begun a treatment study focused on affective and cognitive strategies to help in maintaining weight loss [25]. Cooper et al. have written a book on cognitive-behavioral treatment of obesity [25]. Another book in the popular press is called *The Solution* and focuses on the affective and cognitive aspects of maintaining weight loss [26].

In the book *The Solution*, the author, Laurel Mellin, focuses on feelings, and stresses that it is okay to have both negative and positive feelings. The target should be the way we deal with feelings. This chapter reviews new theories coupled with the need for additional research and what we might do to improve weight loss maintenance.

When we begin placing feelings at the center of the goal to change lifestyle, several steps occur [26]. First helping the patient to ask the simple question "How do I feel?" is important. Mellin indicates that tagging feelings should become a common occurrence happening several times a day. Identifying true feelings allows the patient to find a more appropriate coping strategy than overeating or eating in the absence of hunger.

As the question "How do I feel?" is asked. Identifying feelings, even the difficult ones, is valuable to learning coping skills. This look inside is a beginning to solving the problem of using food as a feeling pacifier. Some of what makes identifying feelings difficult is the fact that it is normal to have many feelings and that often they can be opposite in nature. In MI, identifying the positive and negative aspects of making a change can involve this assessment of feelings.

As with all counseling, there is no perfect path for everyone. Some patients might take longer to recognize a feeling. If a feeling is not recognized immediately, it will occur again in the future.

Mellin's concept of separating feelings from thoughts is important. "I am stressed" is a thought, not a feeling. "I feel angry, sad, and guilty because a coworker indicated that I was inefficient in completing my work today" is a feeling statement. Mellin also describes our ability to eliminate the process of tagging a feeling by identifying smokescreens such as "I feel stressed" and "I feel upset." She urges continuing exploration of the true feelings behind the smokescreens [26].

A way of balancing feelings is to find the opposites in a tagged feeling. Mellin describes this as the "hint of anger behind the calm" or the "joy that bubbles up through depression" [26].

The key to eliminating maladaptive coping strategies and replacing them with appropriate coping strategies is rearranging the way, for example, that sadness is approached to blunt its effect. Instead of eating unhealthy foods in response to sadness, target an appropriate coping strategy — crying. Also, Mellin stresses being skilled in tagging a feeling and then letting it fade. She describes this act of going inside to target feelings as a nurturing process [26].

While we have these new methods with potential strategies, no studies have been published evaluating a behavioral weight loss approach modified to better address affective and cognitive antecedents to unhealthy weight control behaviors. There is related research testing two theories that may prove helpful in maintaining weight loss. The first, Dialectical Behavior Therapy (DBT), is a cognitive behavioral treatment initially used in treating persons with borderline personality disorder. In initial studies, researchers have applied it to the treatment of binge-eating disorder [27, 28]. This theoretical approach uses skills training in distress tolerance and emotion regulation [29]. Telch and his colleagues used this theoretical construct when treating persons with binge-eating disorders [27, 29]. After training in DBT skills, women in this study did not have decreased negative affective behaviors, specifically, but increased their ability to stop behaviors such as binge eating. This research indicates that DBT reduces the urge to eat when experiencing negative affect as opposed to specifically decreasing the negative affect episodes experienced [28]. This means that, for the person who is experiencing sadness over a difficult work-related situation that precedes an eating binge, skills to deal with this sadness will not eliminate the feeling but will provide strategies to eliminate the binge eating behavior. Using DBT skills will allow that feeling of sadness to remain without it being followed by unhealthy eating behaviors.

A second theoretical construct includes the concept of distress tolerance [30]. Distress tolerance is an innovative treatment approach that uses strategies that maintain behavior changes, such as healthy eating habits, even though negative affect exists [30]. At the heart of this concept is the principle of Acceptance and Commitment Therapy (ACT). In this theoretical construct, skills training is provided to manage affective distress without using maladaptive coping responses such as eating unhealthy foods. Skills training is aimed at teaching the obese person to react differently to negative affect. The goal is to break the link between affective distress and the usual maladaptive coping behavior. In this case, the negative affect itself is not the target for change but rather the positive coping strategy used to deal with it. For example, the feeling of being very tired after a difficult day at work might usually be followed by eating a large bag of potato chips. Finding a strategy to break that cycle of feeling tired and immediately eating is the goal. The obese person should be allowed to take time to decide what behavior might follow that tired feeling to allow for a noncalorie remedy such as drinking a glass of water, going on a walk, reading a novel, or calling a friend, for example.

Both distress tolerance and emotion regulation are also key components of DBT [27, 28]. Hayes et al. have written a text on mindfulness and acceptance including DBT and ACT as the conceptual foundation [31].

13.3 THE COUNSELOR-PATIENT INTERACTION

Finally, an important element in counseling is the way the counselor-patient interaction is perceived by both parties. New theories often place counselor and patient on an equal plane. Much of the education in health sciences emphasizes the need for the nutrition counselor to be separate and different from the patient. As nutrition counselors we are expected to be wiser, more professional, more balanced, and more experienced with greater ego strength. The nutrition counselor is in the role of the person who knows how to live a healthy lifestyle. The patient is the student who must learn from the teacher, the nutrition counselor. To be on an equal level with a patient means that the nutrition counselor has failed in some way, when just the opposite is true. Although the nutrition counselor has one level of knowledge, without the specific knowledge the patient brings to the counseling session, forward movement toward lifestyle change is impossible. Taking the position of the importance of including the patient in decision making during a nutrition counseling session has a major effect on the nutrition counselor and patient relationship. It allows for normalization of problems. Problems that the individual patient sees as unique become universal issues. In most nutrition counselor-patient situations the nutrition counselor is seen as strong and the patient weak. "I will help you change your nutrition lifestyle." Instead, the nutrition counselor is willing to normalize what the patient is saying without ducking, despairing, rescuing, or running away.

In summary, research on new theories that include the addition of feelings relative to eating habits can play a large part in nutrition lifestyle change. The concept that the nutrition counselor and the patient are on equal footing working together as a team is also an important new direction needing more exploration in research studies.

REFERENCES

1. Baucom, D.H. and Aiken, P.A., Effect of depressed mood on eating among obese and nonobese dieting and nondieting persons, *J. Personality Soc. Psychol.*, 41, 577–585, 1981.
2. Schotte, D.E., Cools, J., and McNally, R.J., Film-induced negative affect triggers overeating in restrained eaters, *J. Abnormal Psychol.*, 99, 317–320, 1990.

3. Cools, J., Schotte, D.E., and McNally, R.J., Emotional arousal and overeating in restrained eaters, *J. Abnormal Psychol.,* 101, 348–351, 1990.

4. Fitzgibbon, M.L., Stolley, M.R., and Kirschenbaum, D.S., Obese people who seek treatment have different characteristics than those who do not seek treatment, *Health Psychol.,* 12, 342–345, 1993.

5. Geliebter, A. and Aversa, A., Emotional eating in overweight, normal weight, and underweight individuals, *Eating Behav.,* 3, 341–347, 2003.

6. Schlundt, D.G. and Zimering, R.T., The dieter's inventory of eating temptations: a measure of weight control competence, *Addictive Behav.,* 13, 151–164, 1988.

7. Stunkard, A.J. and Messick, S., The Three-Factor Eating Questionnaire to measure dietary restraint, disinhibition and hunger, *J. Psychosomatic Res.,* 13, 151–164, 1988.

8. Stunkard, A.J. and Messick, S., *Eating Inventory Manual,* San Antonio, TX: Harcourt Brace Jovanovich, 1988.

9. Grilo, C.M., Shiffman, S., and Wing, R.R., Relapse crises and coping among dieters, *J. Consulting Clin. Psychol.,* 57, 488–495, 1989.

10. Drapkin, R.G., Wing, R.R., and Shiffman, S., Responses to hypothetical high risk situations: do they predict weight loss in a behavioral treatment program or the context of dietary lapses?, *Health Psychol.,* 14, 427–434, 1995.

11. Karlsson, J., Hallgren, P., Kral, J.G., Lindross, A.K., Sjostrom, L., and Sullivan, M., Predictors and effects of long-term dieting on mental well-being and weight loss in obese women, *Appetite,* 23, 15–26, 1994.

12. Carels, R.A., Hoffman, J., Collins, A., Raber, A.C., Cacciapaglia, H., and O'Brien, W.H., Ecological momentary assessment of temptation and lapse in dieting, *Eating Behav.,* 2, 307–321, 2001.

13. Carels, R.A., Douglass, O.M., Cacciapaglia, H., and O'Brien, W.H., An ecological momentary assessment of relapse crisis in dieting, *J. Consulting Clin. Psychol.,* 72, 341–348, 2004.

14. Byrne, S.M., Copper, A., and Fairburn, C., Weight maintenance and relapse in obesity: a qualitative study, *Intl. J. Obesity,* 27, 955–962, 2003.

15. Byrne, S.M., Copper, A., and Fairburn, C.G., Psychological predictors of weight regain in obesity, *Behav. Res. Ther.,* 42, 1341–1356, 2004.

16. Roberts, R.E., Kaplan, G.A., Shema, S.J., and Strawbridge, W.J., Are the obese at greater risk for depression?, *Am. J. Epidemiol.,* 152, 163–170, 2000.

17. Roberts, R.E., Strawbridge, W.J., Deleger, S., and Kaplan, G.A., Are the fat more jolly? *Ann. Behav. Med.,* 24, 169–180, 2002.

18. Palinkas, L.A., Wingard, D.L., and Barrett-Connor, E., Depressive symptoms in overweight and obese older adults: a test of the "jolly fat" hypothesis, *J. Psychosomatic Res.,* 40, 59–66, 1996.

19. Carpenter, K.M., Hasin, D.S., Allison, D.B., and Faith, M.S., Relationships between obesity and DSM-IV major depressive disorder, suicide ideation, and suicide attempts: results from a general population study, *Am. J. Public Health,* 90, 251–257, 2000.

20. Siegel, J.M., Hyg, M.S., Yancey, A.K., and McCarthy, W.J., Overweight and depressive symptoms among African-American women, *Prev. Med.,* 31, 232–240, 2000.

21. Roberts, R.E., Deleger, S., Strawbridge, W.J., and Kaplan, G.A., Prospective association between obesity and depression: evidence from the Alameda County Study, *Intl. J. Obesity,* 27, 514–521, 2003.

22. Noppa, H. and Hallstrom, T., Weight gain in adulthood in relation to socio-economic factors, mental illness, and personality traits: a prospective study of middle-aged women, *J. Psychosomatic Res.*, 25, 83–89, 1981.

23. DiPietro, L., Anda, R.F., Williamson, D.F., and Stunkard, A.J., Depressive symptoms and weight change in a national cohort of adults, *Intl. J. Obesity*, 16, 745–753, 1992.

24. Korkeila, M., Kaprio, J., Rissanen, A., Koskenvuo, M., and Sorensen, T.A., Predictors of major weight gain in adult Finns: Stress, life satisfaction and personality traits, *Intl. J. Obesity Related Metabolic Disorders*, 22, 949–957, 1998.

25. Cooper, Z., Fairburn, C.G., and Hawker, D.M., *Cognitive-Behavioral Treatment of Obesity: A Clinician's Guide*, New York: The Guilford Press, 2003.

26. Mellin, L., *The Solution*, New York: Harper Collins, 1997, 158–161.

27. Telch, C.F., Agras, W.S., and Linehan, M.M., Group dialectical behavior therapy for binge-eating disorder: a preliminary, uncontrolled trial, *Behav. Ther.*, 31, 569–582, 2000.

28. Telch, C.F., Agras, W.S., and Linehan, M.M., Dialectical behavior therapy for binge eating disorder, *J. Consulting Clin. Psychol.*, 69, 1061–1065, 2001.

29. Linehan, M.M., *Cognitive-Behavioral Treatment of Borderline Personality Disorder*, New York: The Guilford Press, 1993.

30. Brown, R.A., Lejeuz, L.W., Kahler, C.W., Strong, D.R., and Zvolensky, M.J., Distress tolerance and early smoking lapse, *Clin. Psychol. Rev.*, 25(6), 713–733, 2005.

31. Hayes, S.C., Follette, V.M., and Linehan, M.M., *Mindfulness and Acceptance: Expanding the Cognitive Behavioral Tradition*, New York: Guilford Publications, 2004.

14

SUMMARY

This text was devised to use research as a basis for our work with patients and their eventual nutrition lifestyle change. The goal was to provide realistic ways of changing dietary behaviors. We have much to learn relative to predictors of nutrition lifestyle change, but we also have many intervention-related concepts that point to ways in which we can achieve change.

Use of social cognitive theory and stages of change theory are discussed in this text with examples of ways to use each in maximizing the potential for nutrition lifestyle change. The patient-centered counseling is intuitive and often commonsense oriented. It focuses on the individual in whom the nutrition counselor is trying to facilitate change. Scripts in this text provide a road map to follow in working with patients where they are the focus. Figure 14.1 provides a summary of how a dietary intervention might occur. The counseling strategies discussed in previous chapters are presented in this concise diagram.

New research is needed in the area of emotions and the role they play in maintaining nutrition lifestyle change. The concept of internal disinhibition is discussed and may provide a methodology to use in helping persons who relapse because of feelings that trigger inappropriate eating behaviors and to use in forming appropriate coping mechanisms. Teaching skills in changing coping methods can be a key to nutrition lifestyle change.

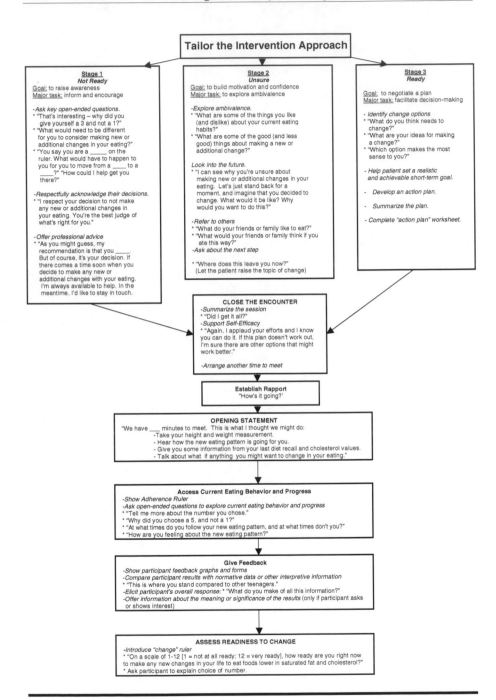

Tailor the Intervention Approach

Stage 1
Not Ready
Goal: to raise awareness
Major task: inform and encourage

- *Ask key open-ended questions.*
  * "That's interesting – why did you give yourself a 3 and not a 1?"
  * "What would need to be different for you to consider making new or additional changes in your eating?"
  * "You say you are a _____ on the ruler. What would have to happen to you for you to move from a _____ to a _____?" "How could I help get you there?"

- *Respectfully acknowledge their decisions.*
  * "I respect your decision to not make any new or additional changes in your eating. You're the best judge of what's right for you."

- *Offer professional advice*
  * "As you might guess, my recommendation is that you _____. But of course, it's your decision. If there comes a time soon when you decide to make any new or additional changes with your eating, I'm always available to help. In the meantime, I'd like to stay in touch.

Stage 2
Unsure
Goal: to build motivation and confidence
Major task: to explore ambivalence

- *Explore ambivalence.*
  * "What are some of the things you like (and dislike) about your current eating habits?"
  * "What are some of the good (and less good) things about making a new or additional change?"

Look into the future.
  * "I can see why you're unsure about making new or additional changes in your eating. Let's just stand back for a moment, and imagine that you decided to change. What would it be like? Why would you want to do this?"

- *Refer to others*
  * "What do your friends or family like to eat?"
  * "What would your friends or family think if you ate this way?"
  -*Ask about the next step*

  * "Where does this leave you now?"
  (Let the patient raise the topic of change)

Stage 3
Ready
Goal: to negotiate a plan
Major task: facilitate decision-making

- *Identify change options*
  * "What do you think needs to change?"
  * "What are your ideas for making a change?"
  * "Which option makes the most sense to you?"

- *Help patient set a realistic and achievable short-term goal.*

- *Develop an action plan.*

- *Summarize the plan.*

- *Complete "action plan" worksheet.*

CLOSE THE ENCOUNTER
-*Summarize the session*
* "Did I get it all?"
-*Support Self-Efficacy*
* "Again, I applaud your efforts and I know you can do it. If this plan doesn't work out, I'm sure there are other options that might work better."

-*Arrange another time to meet*

Establish Rapport
"How's it going?"

OPENING STATEMENT
"We have ___ minutes to meet. This is what I thought we might do:
-Take your height and weight measurement.
- Hear how the new eating pattern is going for you.
- Give you some information from your last diet recall and cholesterol values.
- Talk about what if anything you might want to change in your eating."

Access Current Eating Behavior and Progress
-*Show Adherence Ruler*
-*Ask open-ended questions to explore current eating behavior and progress*
* "Tell me more about the number you chose."
* "Why did you choose a 5, and not a 1?"
* "At what times do you follow your new eating pattern, and at what times don't you?"
* "How are you feeling about the new eating pattern?"

Give Feedback
-*Show participant feedback graphs and forms*
-*Compare participant results with normative data or other interpretive information*
* "This is where you stand compared to other teenagers."
-*Elicit participant's overall response:* * "What do you make of all this information?"
-*Offer information about the meaning or significance of the results (only if participant asks or shows interest)*

ASSESS READINESS TO CHANGE
-*Introduce "change" ruler*
* "On a scale of 1-12 [1 = not at all ready; 12 = very ready], how ready are you right now to make any new changes in your life to eat foods lower in saturated fat and cholesterol?"
* Ask participant to explain choice of number.

Figure 14.1 Dietary intervention summary. (Courtesy of Steven Malcolm Berg Smith, M.S.)

Appendix A

WHAT YOUR BABY CAN DO AND HOW AND WHAT TO FEED HIM

Age	Developmental Landmarks	Feeding Suggestions
Birth to 6 months	Sucks Roots for nipple Swallows liquids	Breast milk Iron-fortified infant formula
5 to 7 months	Holds neck steady Sits with or without support Follows food with eyes Opens mouth when food is offered Draws in lower lip when spoon is removed Begins to swallow thickened food	Iron-fortified infant cereal Rice (start with first) Barley Mix with breast milk or iron-fortified infant cereal. Feed with spoon. Breast milk/iron-fortified infant formula
6 to 8 months	Sits without support Moves tongue to side Chews food with up and down motion Reaches for and palms food (palmar grasp) Begins finger feeding Begins drinking from a cup	Well-cooked, mashed vegetables and fruits Sticky rice Unsweetened wheat-free dry cereals Corn tortilla strips Breast milk/iron-fortified infant formula

Age	What Your Baby Can Do	What to Feed Him
7 to 10 months	Bites off pieces of food Rotary chewing pattern Moves food from side to side in mouth Forms lips to cup Pincer grasp (thumb and forefinger) develops	Cooked or canned vegetables and fruits, chopped Cheese, cut up Cooked beans, mashed Pasta, cut into pieces Unsweetened dry cereals with wheat Toast squares, crackers, tortilla strips Breast milk/iron-fortified infant formula
9 to 12 months	Improved pincer grasp Greater interest in solid foods Drinks from covered toddler cup without assistance	Soft cooked and raw foods, cut up Egg yolks, mashed Cheese, cut up Soft meats, fish, or poultry chopped Casseroles with any large pieces cut up Unsweetened dry cereals, toast, crackers Breast milk/iron-fortified infant formula
12 months and beyond	Becomes more skillful at self-feeding Begins to use a spoon Increased sociability in regards to eating	Soft table foods Whole eggs Whole pasteurized milk

Modified from Kleinman, R.E., Ed., *Pediatric Nutrition Handbook*, 5th ed., American Academy of Pediatrics, 2004.

Appendix B

PARENTAL FEEDING PRACTICES INTERVENTION SESSION #1 — OVERHEADS

SESSION #1: INTERVENTION GROUP OVERHEADS

Parents influence a child's behavior by ...

- **Parental Modeling:** Your own eating behavior. Example: You drink milk every evening with dinner.
- **Food Environment:** The foods you make available to eat. Example: You buy applesauce and bananas every week to have at home to eat.
- **Feeding Practices:** How you offer food or react to your child's food intake patterns

Your infant is a unique individual, and if you handle feeding sensitively, you are helping your child to grow up to be a happy and healthy person.

People feel about eating and react to eating in many different ways that are all normal and acceptable and successful. You will be safe going along with your child's eating behaviors, however odd they might seem.

Feeding with a Division of Responsibility

You are responsible for what your child is offered to eat and the way in which it is offered.

She is responsible for how much of it she eats, and even whether she eats.

Parents are responsible for what is given to eat and the way in which it is presented:

- Choose food that your child can handle, such as the right textures, so she can control it in her mouth and swallow it as well as possible; for example, starting cooked or canned fruits and vegetables first. Also, you are responsible for what kinds of food are given, such as a variety of fruits and vegetables.
- Hold your baby on your lap or support her in an upright position to introduce solids so she can explore her food. She'll be braver about trying new foods.
- Have her sit up straight and face forward. She'll be able to swallow better and will be less likely to choke.
- Talk to her in a quiet and encouraging manner while she eats. Don't entertain her or overwhelm her with attention, but do keep her company.

Children are responsible for how much and whether to eat.

- Wait for him to pay attention to each spoonful before you try to feed it to him.
- Let him touch his food — in the dish, on the spoon. You wouldn't eat something if you didn't know anything about it, would you?
- Feed at his tempo. Don't try to get him to go faster or slower than he wants to. Look into his eyes during the feeding process so you can share this experience with him.
- Allow him to feed himself with his fingers as soon as he shows interest.
- Stop feeding when he indicates he has had enough (turns head away, pushes plate or spoon away, won't open mouth).

Children want to grow. They have built within them the need to get better at everything they do. Eating is no exception.

Appendix C

PARENTAL FEEDING PRACTICES INTERVENTION SESSION #2 — HANDOUTS

SESSION #2: INTERVENTION GROUP HANDOUTS

Feeding Your Baby Fruits and Vegetables

Do ...

- Use cooked or canned fruits or vegetables at first. The heating process makes them less likely to cause allergic reactions.
- Include fruits like those that are canned in water, juice, or syrup and then drained. Put the fruit through a baby-food grinder, mash it, chop it, or cut it into small pieces depending on your baby's ability to gum and swallow.
- Offer raw fruits such as peaches, pears, and plums once they have been eaten in their cooked form. Remove all skin and chop into small pieces.
- Save time by giving your baby the cooked vegetables you are having at meals. Like fruit, put the vegetable through a baby-food grinder, mash it, chop it, or cut it into small pieces depending on your baby's ability to gum and swallow.
- Offer one new food at a time. Wait 2 to 3 days before adding another new food to check for allergic reactions.
- Adjust serving sizes for your child's age. In general, figure a serving equals 1 tablespoon of food per year of age. So a serving for a 1-year-old would be 1 tablespoon.

- Serve a variety of fruits and vegetables at meals and snacks. By the time your baby is 9 to 12 months of age, he needs a minimum of 2 servings of fruit and 3 servings of vegetables, or 5 servings from the fruit and vegetable group combined, to have a healthy diet.

Feeding Your Baby Fruits and Vegetables

Don't ...

- Offer your baby unlimited juice. While some juice is fine, too much can lead to cavities and leave your baby too full for other foods. Choose a juice that is a good form of vitamin C, such as orange or grapefruit, or one that is fortified with vitamin C. Offer juice at snack times only, in a cup not a bottle. Limit juice to half a cup a day at first. If your baby wants more, dilute it with water to make it go further.
- Feed your baby certain home-prepared vegetables such as beets, carrots, collard greens, spinach, and turnips when they are less than 6 months of age.
- Feel you must use commercial baby foods. Commercial baby foods are OK to use, but they are not really needed. When buying commercial baby foods, read the label. Avoid those that have water as the main ingredient and contain a lot of carbohydrate fillers such as starches.
- Feed your baby fruits or vegetables that she could choke on. Foods that are unsafe include raw apple, carrot, or celery pieces. Also, avoid whole grapes or cherry tomatoes — cut them into quarters instead.
- Be alarmed if you notice changes in your baby's stools after starting fruits and vegetables. It is normal for stools to change colors. It is also normal to see small lumps of food in your baby's stools.

DIVISIONS OF RESPONSIBILITY

Parents are responsible for what is given to eat and the way in which it is presented:

- Choose food that your child can handle, such as the right textures, so she can control it in her mouth and swallow it as well as possible; for example, starting cooked or canned fruits and vegetables first. Also, you are responsible for what kinds of food are given, such as a good variety of fruits and vegetables.

- Hold your baby on your lap or support her in an upright position to introduce solids so she can explore her food. She'll be braver about trying new foods.
- Have her sit up straight and face forward. She'll be able to swallow better and be less likely to choke.
- Talk to her in a quiet and encouraging manner while she eats. Don't entertain her or overwhelm her with attention but do keep her company.

Children are responsible for how much and whether to eat.

- Wait for him to pay attention to each spoonful before you try to feed it to him.
- Let him touch his food — in the dish, on the spoon. You wouldn't eat something if you didn't know anything about it, would you?
- Feed at his tempo. Don't try to get him to go faster or slower than he wants to. Look into his eyes during the feeding process so you can share this experience with him.
- Allow him to feed himself with his fingers as soon as he shows interest.
- Stop feeding when he indicates he has had enough (turns head away, pushes plate or spoon away, won't open mouth).

FEEDING BEHAVIOR WORKSHEET

Parental Modeling

What vegetables do I eat that my child will see me eat?
What fruits do I eat that my child will see me eat?

Food Environment

What vegetables do I *not* like but know are important for good health and will start to buy and offer to my child?
When will I offer these?
What fruits do I *not* like but know are important for good health and will start to buy and offer?
When will I offer these?

Feeding Practices

What is one feeding practice that I will work on?

INDEX

Printed and bound by CPI Group (UK) Ltd, Croydon, CR0 4YY

17/10/2024

01775691-0004